Mind Force Se

By A. Thomas Perhacs

Published by Velocity Group Publishing

PO Box 9516 Hamilton, NJ 08650 www.advancedmindpower.com www.mindforcesecrets.com

Introduction

DISCLAIMER

Neither A. Thomas Perhacs nor Velocity Group Publishing assumes any responsibility for the use or misuse of the concepts, methods and strategies contained in this book. The reader is warned that the use of some or all of the techniques in this book may result in legal consequences, civil and/or criminal.

USE OF THIS BOOK IS DONE AT YOUR OWN RISK.

(Updated Version, August 2008)

When I first wrote the material in this book, I considered it to be quite a bit different than most of the other works I had seen in the market, and I wondered if I even wanted to publish the material. I did extensive research finding out how a lot of these things work through my own experiences and those of students, colleagues and friends I have met over the years. This book actually contains three (3) of my most popular manuscripts:

The Magneto Method

Mind Portal

Internal Power Centers

I believe the information in this manual is fresh and will allow you to begin to understand yet another facet of your mind power.

The mind is all encompassing and yet, it is as powerful as we make it. This book covers ground which most people would cast off as being strange or weird. Had I not experienced a lot of the concepts covered in this manuscript, I would feel the same way.

Most who have read this works have claimed they were some of the best books they have read and in fact answered a lot of their questions. I hope you will find it to be the same for you. Enjoy this book as the insights are interesting…To say the least…

A Thomas Perhacs

Hamilton, New Jersey

August, 2008

Table Of Contents

3

Mind Force Attraction: The Magneto Method

By A. Thomas Perhacs

Published by Velocity Group Publishing

PO Box 9516 Hamilton, NJ 08650   www.advancedmindpower.com   www.mindforcesecrets.com

CHAPTER 1: Creating a Powerful Energy Source

How you can create a potent energy that will allow your attraction abilities to increase substantially

magneto- \Mag"net*o-\ [See <u>Magnet</u>.] A prefix meaning pertaining to, produced by, or in some way connected with, magnetism. (2) Permanent-magnet alternating generator employed when the output of energy required is very small. Magnetic Field.

Most people would wonder why they would want to be more magnetic with their energy…Most people would ask, does this really work? What is it about some people that can attract to them virtually any thing that they want?

What you will find in this course are practical methods to increase your energy and attraction power. These methods do in fact work and can work for you, if you apply them to your current situation. You will learn methods that until recently have been regarded as secret methods of energy & attraction development.

There are many examples of how this works, but what is not usually explained is how you can harness this power for your own purposes. We are going to take a look into this unique topic and really dissect what it takes to become the type of person that can positively attract things to them. Here are some examples

Examples of Magnetism and Energy Manipulation

- o **Rock Stars:** Did you ever notice how girls will throw themselves at a musical performer? They are literally in a trance that the performer has put them in through the musical vibration and the lyrics of the songs.
- o **Preachers:** Ever been to a powerful sermon, where the congregation gets up out of their chairs to conduct healing or highly spiritual prayer sessions?
- o **Motivational Speakers:** The motivational speaker entices his crowd by getting them to do what he wants them to do (at least for the moment). He can sell them books, tapes and additional seminar tickets and they do what ever he/she says.

11

- **High Powered Business People:** How do you think someone becomes a millionaire or multi-millionaire? More often times than naught, they are the type of people that can get people to do things for the company than they would ever do for themselves, thus allowing them to benefit greatly from the growth of the company.

What you will notice in each of the cases above is that each of these types of people has a powerful attraction energy mechanism that goes on between them and their respective audiences. This magnetic energy is within all of us. What these people do is harness it to attract to them what they want.

We will be studying in detail exactly what it takes to attract anything that you want in your life as long as you keep in mind that you must do it with the goal of making it a win/win. Which means your attraction should not only be a benefit for you but for your subject as well.

Expectations

So, what can you expect from this course? You can expect that the path will be uncovered for you to learn how to increase your energy and become a powerful attracting force. The caveat is that these types of things take time and effort to learn, and that merely reading or listening to CD is not going to make you a "Magneto".

You must put action behind the concepts discussed and make the effort to want to change. Once you realize that in life, change is a constant and that you must change for the better in order to get this to work, you will naturally understand the full potential and how powerfully the concepts in this course can work for you.

"Change is the only constant in life. Come to terms with change and you can excel at anything in your life"

Magnetic/Internal Energy

This course will go into great detail on how to create the physical aspect of energy Manipulation as well as great detail on how to harness and increase the Mental Power Training that is "Magneto". Here is a brief explanation of the different types of energy.

- **Physical Energy**- This is the physical manifestation of the energy that you have inside of your body. This requires training that will enable you to produce an actual feeling to your energy versus just using your mind.
- **Mental Energy**- Using the mind alone to produce the results that you are looking for.
- **Sexual Energy**- The energy that can be used to super charge your magnetism.

Naturally, using both the physical and mental aspects of this will cause your energy manipulation results to go up exponentially.

Everyone has a certain amount of energy that they have developed over their years and to some extent, like some athletes are naturally more gifted than others, there are some that have a pre-disposition on how to use their energy abilities to their maximum than others.

This being the case, some of you will already be at higher level than others. Just know that no matter where you are on the scale, this course will teach you how to improve your ability to use your energy.

You can use this energy for many different things, such as healing or helping people or for combative or self-defense measures. Although these may be the most common, there are probably hundreds if not thousands of techniques that can be used with energy.

When you wonder how real this magnetic energy is, just remember some of the examples listed above as well other examples that you can find if you do the research. A lot of times, when you undertake training like this, you need to do the proper research to make sure you are justified in your endeavor.

" You must feed your mind the outcomes that you want, not the ones that you don't want"

BREATHING WITH POWER:

Often when new practitioners begin doing energy Power Exercises, they will overlook the most vital information in this book: how to breathe correctly.

After you have fully read the book, and listened to the CDs, you will have a very good understanding of how all of this works. You can't learn the art of focus without it!

In order to be able to attract with power, you need a power source. In fact there are several power sources we will tap into. One of them is our breath, the other is our mental power. Gaining control over your breathing is an important step in gaining control over yourself.

You can't live without breath, and yet how many people breathe the correct way?

Your breath can be a source of power if you know how to harness that power. What I want you to learn how to do is to breathe from your diaphram not your chest. Many people breathe from their chest, when this is the worst way to breath.

Babies breathe through their bellys, and so should you. We call this belly breathing. In order to become proficient at this type of breathing you will want to focus on breathing from your diaphram. We will cover much more of this in the in the Mind Force Meditation training, but start to think about how you breathe and notice if you are breathing through your chest or through your belly.

Energy Vibrations

Everything that we do Vibrates… All energy vibrations are related to both animate and inanimate objects. This vibrational energy is one of the many types of energy that we are going to cultivate to develop our attraction powers.

Anything that produces light is a transmitter. It produces light energy. Light is energy…. The complete field or continuum of energy covers all the vibrations that an object will respond to, or has within it.

Each of the vibrations of our senses responds and combines with specific frequencies. It detects and vibrates with these frequencies. It repels some of these frequencies, and it absorbs some of these frequencies. When your sensing faculty detects a frequency, some of it is absorbed and some is repelled. The frequency that is absorbed is converted to a different frequency, which is then transmitted to the brain.

All senses receive energy from the electromagnetic field, convert it to nerve energy, and transmit it to the brain. The sense of sight receives light energy, converts it to nerve energy, and transmits it to the brain. The same can be said of the sense of smell, sense of taste, touch, and hearing. Our biological senses detect physical vibrations, convert them, and transmit them to the left-brain hemisphere.

The left-brain hemisphere receives nerve energy from the physical senses, converts it to subjective energy, and transmits it to the right brain hemisphere.

The right brain hemisphere also has a set of senses. They are subjective, at a different dimension, not within the physical electromagnetic spectrum that includes sound vibrations, visible light, etc.

By understanding how this vibrational energy works is important so that you can start to experience the value of taking conscious thoughts and feeding them into the sub-consious or un-consious mind. All of this directly relates to becoming a magneto…

When things vibrate, and we sense information through the internal vibrations of an object we can then start to create a higher understanding of how we can then relate to that vibration in terms of its power, clarity, information, feelings etc.

" Ideas are your masters and determine your attitude"

Exercise: Sensing Vibes(vibration) Next time you meet someone do this exercise. It can be someone you know or a complete stranger.

1. When you meet them and shake their hand or greet them start to feel their energy vibrations.
2. Determine in your own mind before they tell you how they are doing, what their feelings are.
   a. Are they upset
   b. Are they happy
   c. Are the feeling good or bad
   d. Are their relationships stable
   e. Any other feelings that they may have
3. See if you can then project your good feelings on them and get them to notice by them

telling you how positive or good you feel to them today.

Your body's vibrations penetrate objects within your presence and affect the internal vibrations of the objects. Your body radiation charges up the object with your own frequencies. This is why often times you can tell how someone is doing just by the "vibes" that they are putting off.

When you touch a ring, or another personal item that you have for instance, it becomes an extension of you; it is saturated with your own vibrations. Later, someone else can hold the object, and sense the vibrations of the previous owner. Of course it takes great sensitivity to do this, and you can learn this with a little practice.

Exercise: Object Sensitivity

1. Take a personal object from someone you know
2. Hold it and start to feel the energy of the person
3. Do your best to tell something about the person

You can also try multiple items from different people and try and feel whose item the object is. Make it a game and this will be great fun as you are learning how to become more sensitive from someone's vibrational energy.

"Always Discipline Your Imagination"

CHAPTER 2: Attraction Energy and the Emotions

When you fully understand the connection between your magnetic attraction energy and your emotions, you will truly have the answer to attracting those things you want.

The law of attraction, attracts to you everything you need according to the nature of your thought life. Your environment and financial condition are perfect reflections of your habitual thinking…..**THOUGHT RULES THE WORLD!**

"There is no shortage of what you want, It is like the air you breath"

Once you truly understand that everything that you desire is out their waiting for you, you will get excited about the possibilities of what life has in store for you.

The problem with most people, is they think too small, or their expectations are set too low. They don't really believe they can have what they desire, and so therefore they get what they are attracting through their energy…Which is shortage and lack.

Just come to the conclusion that everything you want is out there and has your name attached to it. Begin to really and truly believe that the creative attraction power within you is unlimited….. **So believe it……**

The Steps to Begin Becoming a Powerful Attracting Force

- **Becoming an Attracting Force (Drawing things to you):** This is the totality of what Magneto is all about. Getting yourself to become an attracting force, a mechanism to draw to you what you want, need and desire.

- **Physical Energy:** Fully comprehending that the attraction force is a totally physical force that you can increase and mold to any given situation.

- **Mental Energy:** The mental side of the game is the side that takes most work. Getting our mind to function as we want it to, not as it has functioned up until now.

- **Sexual Energy:** Harnessing the most potent energy we have to utilize in the attraction process. There is no more powerful attraction than that of the pulling of sexual energy.

- **Energy Vibrations:** Learning how to get the right vibrations sent out to get the things you desire. The key is to make sure you are sending out the right positive vibrations for the desired effect.

- **Seeing yourself as a "Magneto":** See yourself as a powerful magneto or attraction force. Believing that you are that Magneto is important.

- **Alpha Male/Female:** In relationships or looking for romance, are you playing the role as the alpha, the first or the leader. This is a mind set that transfers to the physical as well as the sexual.

The Seven (7) Positive Emotions

These are the emotions you want to be cultivating at all times. In order to keep yourself going towards the objectives of what you want, you must be in a place mentally that is positive and leads to a robust well being.

1. Desire
2. Faith
3. Love
4. Sex
5. Enthusiasm
6. Romance
7. Hope

"Don't ever let anyone ruin your day or spoil your attitude of fun"

18

The Nine (9) Mental Impurities to Avoid

1. Envy
2. Hatred
3. Revenge
4. Covetousness
5. Superstition
6. Anger
7. Fear
8. Worry
9. Jealousy

These (9) mental impurities should be removed from your life as much as possible as they have no positive value.

Anytime you feel one of these emotions creeping in, you must recall the power of negative and these mental impurities. Negative is 14 times stronger than positive, so if you decide to harness one of these emotions, you may be causing an amplification of the wrong emotions, thus causing problems to occur in your life.

The good news, is you control your emotions more than you think. Don't ever let someone or something control your emotions. First off, no one can control your emotions, you must decide to let them.

With these skills, you are now becoming a different person, a stronger person with a stronger mind and the ability to negate the negative in your life.

Affirmation: "I have a strong mind and can control my thoughts and emotions."

Chapter 3: Advanced Mind Power Training

Discarding your past mistakes, failures and baggage is the first step to making your mind, body and spirit clean from past garbage

The Past is Not Your Doorway to Your Future

Probably the most important thing for you to do as you prepare to become a powerful attracting force is to discard your past mistakes and failures. It doesn't matter where you have been in life, it is only important that you, plant your feet and move from where you are.

Most people take all of their past failures and baggage and allow it to effect them now. Whether you were successful in the past or a total loser, failure, geek or whatever terms you want to use.....Dump it.. Get over it.. Like we covered before, change is inevitable so make it positive and change for the better.

"Your dominant mental attitude is your real boss"

The following are mental exercises to perform that will allow you to get better control of yourself by discarding the negatives of the past, while at the same time increasing the vision of past successes.

Exercise: Shrinking your problems and challenges into insignificance

1. Take all of your problems and challenges and put them in a picture frame
2. See them very vividly; almost so that you could touch them, feel them.
3. Slowly start to adjust the picture so that they start to shrink.
4. Shrink them down into the bottom of the frame and then push them all the way over to one side.

De-Focus from them due to them being so insignificant. Once you shrink them down so far, they will be imperceptible by you.

The past never goes away…The subconscious mind stores every event that you have ever experienced. This is why you just can't totally get rid of it, but you can make it so small and insignificant that it no longer affects you.

20

Take out the Trash- Dumping the Garbage of Your Mind

Make a conscious decision to get rid of all of the garbage of your mind. I use the analogy that you need to just take out the trash. The thing is that like all garbage, you need to continually take the garbage out. As you get started, you may find yourself taking the garbage out everyday so that you can keep yourself focused on where you need to go.

So how do you do this? It really is easy, you just need to turn the switch in your mind from lose to win. The subconscious portion of the mind believes what ever you tell it to believe, whether it is true or not. So what you need to do is feed your sub-conscious mind with what you want it to act on, not what you don't want.

"Mind Fasting"- Removing Mental Impurities

Just like you can remove impurities from your body by fasting from food, you can do the same thing with your mind, by allowing yourself to fast from the negative things that get into your mind and abstain from those things for a predetermined period of time.

This could include not watching the news on TV, not reading newspapers, staying away from negative people, physically removing your self from a harmful relationship.

Affirmation: "Opportunities are always knocking on my door"

The Key to Controlling Your Emotional Content

If you truly understand the following statement, this entire book will have been worth you reading. As a matter of fact, this one statement can change your life the moment you internalize it and act on it.....Now

21

> **"It is how you act that determines how you feel, not how you feel that determines how you act".**

Many think that you are controlled by your emotions. In fact, those that become a strong attractor or Controller (see Manipulation Course) decide to make their actions control their emotional content. Action has a positive effect on your emotions because you are creating a habit of doing what needs to be done, not using your emotions as the reason for lack of action.

You are in total control of how you want to feel at any given time. Your emotions are controlled by you, and you alone. Many people will say, "He hurt my feelings". Well that is incorrect, because no one can hurt your feelings. They may say or do something that causes you to react a certain way, but they are by no means controlling how you feel.

Learn how to act the way you want to feel not how outside circumstances are controlling you. This one key is really what this course is all about. Write this statement down on a piece of paper and carry it around with you always. When you feel yourself getting down for some reason, read this powerful sentence and commit it to your memory, it's that powerful……

> **Affirmation: "It is how I act that determines how I feel, not how I feel that determines how I act".**

Balloon Head Exercise

With this exercise, you allow yourself to release negative thoughts and impulses.

1. Sit down in a comfortable chair
2. Close your eyes
3. Take 10 deep breaths, feeling yourself starting to get more relaxed with each breath
4. Visualize a limp, unfilled balloon on the top of your head.
5. Start to fill the balloon up with all of the negative thoughts, problems and challenges that you may have.

22

6. After the balloon is filled, visualize it taking off and going up into the sky and into space.
   Let the problems float off into depths of space, never to return to your line of thinking.

Setting Your Mind Switch to Success

Flip your switch to success. To do this, you must first come up with a definition of what success is for you. It could mean getting in the absolute best shape of your life or achieving a high level of financial success. For others it could mean fulfilling a life long dream to tour a part of the world that you have never seen.

Whatever your definition of success is, just decide that you are going to start to go get it. Many people never attain what they want because they never truly know what THEIR definition of success is. Get your definition of success and then flip the switch!

Getting Your Mind to accept what you want not what you don't want

The next step in the process is to get your mind to accept the powerful new objectives that you want. You must get a clear picture of what you want in order to go towards that direction.

Sometimes you must force the direction of your mind. At first your mind will resist going in the direction you want it to go. Get control of the mind and get it to accept what you want it to. The subconscious mind as stated before, will take any thought or experience and catalog it, whether it is real or imagined.

At first, you will be focusing on where you want to be, not where you are. The mind can be tricked into thinking one way or the other. The thing is you must make sure that your outside physical actions are living up to what you are feeding to the mind.

Putting Your Best Look Forward

Part of creating a powerful attraction force is looking the best that you can. It is not important how you look, but how you carry yourself. As long as you have a strong self-concept of yourself,

23

others will look at you as attractive because you are comfortable with yourself no matter what physical imperfections one might have.

Redirecting the Mind: Focusing on the future that you want to create, not one that is dictated by your past. Again the past doesn't equal your future. Use this to redirect your mind efforts.

✓ Think attraction & that which you want to attract will follow

✓ Think non-attraction & you will get that.

Exercise: Thought images and mental pictures for attracting what you want

1. Focus on what you want

2. Build a picture of that thing

3. Add density and depth to the image

4. Keep it in your mind at all times

Affirmation: " I Attract (Object of Desire) to me like a Magnet"

CHAPTER 4: Creating The Mind Machine: Magneto

The mind is a can be formed into a mechanism for attaining everything you ever wanted in your life.

What is a Mind Machine

A mind machine is mechanism that you can use to create a more powerful attracting force. The mind machine is one that you construct to perform tasks that you need in order to attract certain things to you.

As stated before, the mind is the most powerful tool that you have access to. By creating a mind machine, you are setting perimeters for how you are going to obtain the results that you are looking for.

The magneto can be turned on and off by you, just as you would turn off an appliance. The mind will follow the instructions that you give to it.

How to Create a Mind Machine or Magneto

The mind machine is a personal tool that you create. It is a creative device that you use in order to achieve your goals and objectives. The design is based on how you want it to look and feel.

- **Projector**- Your eyes are the video portion of the projector and your ears are the audio portion. Use this projector to replay how you should have done something better or pre-play a situation in the future.
- **Magneto**- The machine is like a big electro magnet that can bring anything you want into your reality by turning it on and giving it directions and coordinates.
- **Workshop of the Mind**- You build a workshop that only you have access to. You control the entire process of what goes on there.
- **Computer with Editing Board**- You visualize a large computer in front of you that only you have permission to control. You set up certain guidelines for the programming. You also have controls that can increase the following:
    Brightness
    Increase size of picture
    Make images more vivid

How To Use It

You use the Magneto or Mind Machine to attract to you the things that you desire. It becomes a part of you. You control it and it acts on your commands and suggestions.

Most people have similar machines in their mind, the only difference is they use these "mind machines" for self-destructive purposes.

Imagination/Visualization

Exercise- Project & clothe your ideas with intense visibility/Clearness of the image.

1. Start with an image of what you want

2. Start to put meat on the bones of that idea

3. Build it so strong that it is as if it already is happening

4. Future Pace it by seeing it as in your past

5. Mental picture of total fulfillment of your objective

> ## "Build in your mind that which you want to attract"

Visualizing what you want and the 5 different ways to do it

You can find many different ways to visualize, many different exercises and many different interpretations of what visualizing something is. One key point as it relates to visualizing is that some people can visualize more powerfully than others and so they will have a little bit of an edge on the actual visualization process.

Just like any talents that you have, some of you will be able to visualize better due to a better **"minds eye"** that will be able to see the pictures more clearly. Although this is true, what the exercises in this course will do is increase your ability to visualize and see things in a more real way.

There are primarily 5 ways in which to visualize and depending on what you are looking to accomplish will depend on which one you use and for what purpose.

#1 Through Your Own Eyes- This is where you do the visualization with you seeing all of the pictures through your own eyes. You are visualizing this as if you are in the picture.

#2 Seeing Yourself in the Picture- This is where you are seeing your self in the picture from another location. This would be like watching yourself on TV.

#3 Seeing it from above- This is the birds' eye view from above. This allows you to see the image from above and looking down as if you were flying above the picture.

#4 The Television Screen- This is similar to #2, and the only difference is that you actually envision a TV and you have the control over the screen size, volume, brightness and other features.

#5 From someone else's viewpoint- This is where you visualize using someone else's vantage point. This allows you to be able to relate to how someone else may be viewing the situation.

Imagine Abundance/Riches instead of Lack.

Peace instead of Discord

Health instead of Sickness

Prosperity instead of Mediocrity

Love instead of the void of love

Strength instead of weakness

"He calleth the things that are not, as though they were....and the unseen becomes the seen. (Romans 4:17)

Attracting Piano Exercise (Example): The piano can be any object of your desire.

1. You Don't have one to play

2. Visualize one with keys

3. Know that your Subconscious mind will find you one to play

What is the Mindset of an Attractor

- **Controlling thoughts:** Attractors in life learn to control the thoughts in their head by disciplining themselves to only think positive thoughts. If you hold the wrong thought in the mind for too long, it will become manifest just like the good ones will, with the exception that negative thoughts are about 14 times stronger than positive ones.
- **What you think you become (See also "Think and Grow Rich"-Napoleon Hill):** Every thought that you have, fires off a picture of that thought causing your subconscious to focus on the picture for the amount of time you are focused on the thought. If the focus is on "Mind Garbage" or "Mind Candy", it can only cause mixed results.
- **Sex Transmutation:** Learning how to take the physical aspect of sex and turning it into energy for the mind to develop positive habits, disciplines and achievements.

Attraction Power

1. **Faith:** Having that tiny seed so that you can glimpse that which is in the unseen and make it seen.

2. **Receptivity:** Being open to the possibility of the attraction force.

3. **Initiating to contemplate God's riches**: Understanding that God wants you to have whatever you want and that he will bless you based on your ability to deserve it.

"Project to The Future, Live In The Moment"

Principles of Sowing and Reaping

- **How to magnify your blessings:** You magnify your blessing in direct correlation to the amount you give back to the world. As a giver, your mind becomes free to accept the blessings that come from giving.
- **Understanding that your blessings are tied to your effort:** Blessings will come when you put the work in with belief that you are entitled to the blessings that your work has created.
- **Why some sabotage their blessings:** A lot of people feel they are not worthy of blessings based on their perception of what it takes to receive those blessings. Most people put in a sufficient amount of work, but where they fall short is believing that they have not done enough work to receive the blessings. Once you acknowledge your effort the blessings will follow.

Shortage of Blessings

1. **Greed:** You are never satisfied and your lust for more gets in the way of how you received the blessings in the first place.

2. **Selfishness:** Being not willing to share your blessings with others.

3. **Fear:** Instead of being faithful and knowing that more blessings are headed your way, you covet the blessings as if they are the last ones you will ever receive thus causing you to receive that which you fear the most to come to pass.

"Bless others and you will be blessed yourself"

CHAPTER 5: Potent Attraction Techniques:

Unlocking the keys to the Magneto Process

Specific strategies and techniques will allow your mind to associate and build a strong link to the objects you desire to attract.

What the Mind Responds To: When looking to attract someone, these are the key emotional triggers that will bring someone at your request.

- The Desire for Sex Expression
- Love
- A burning desire for fame, power, financial gain, or money
- Music
- Friendship
- Goal alignment with those of a like mind
- Mutual Suffering
- Auto Suggestion/Self Hypnosis
- Fear
- Alcohol and Drugs

> **"The only chance you have is the chance you make for yourself, so decide to make it a successful one."**

Turning on the Magnetic Lasso or Casting Your Attraction Line

Just like a cowboy uses a lasso to bring a calf or bull into his control, you can use an energetic lasso that allows you to visualize pulling someone or something into your space.

The Magnetic Attraction Box

You can also form a box or bubble around the person or thing you are looking to attract. This is a way to place someone into a box of your own design for you own reasons. The stronger you visualize these things the more they will manifest to reality.

Creating an Instant Connection

- **People Want to Get to Know you When they can:**
  - Know You
  - Like You
  - Trust You
- **Breathing for attraction** (Inhale to attract): By using the inhale, you allow your powerful attraction to work in a pulling manner. Your outward breath can repel, but your inhale can attract people, animals or objects.
- **Intent:** Your intent must be that of an attractor, someone that will naturally and easily be able to attract or connect with anyone or anything whenever they desire.
- **Rapport Building:** To attract people, you need to know how to get into rapport with them and create a bond. (See Manipulation for more detail)
- **Modeling:** When you model someone's actions, it allows you to create a commonality with that person, thus causing you to develop a deep level of contact.

Exercise: Thought images and mental pictures for attracting what you want.

1. Focus on what you want

2. Build a picture of that thing

3. Add density and depth to the image

4. Keep it in your mind at all times

Exercise- You are the Distribution Center for Wealth

1. You bestow it on others first

2. Unlimited Inventory

3. You have the right to anything you want if your motive is right

Faith is......The substance of things hoped for, evidence of things not seen (Hebrews 11:1)

FAITH, ZEAL, CONFIDENCE is WEALTH ENTHUSIASM

1. Creative power is in thoughts and feelings

2. Learning to limit circumstances and block them

    a. Impediments

    b. Obstructions

    c. Delays

    d. Obstacles

Powerful Attraction Techniques for:

✓ **Wealth:** Focus not only on the wealth that you want, but the physical aspects to that wealth.
✓ **Romance:** Build the perfect partner in your head first and then let your Mind Machine work to find that perfect partner.
✓ **Good Fortune:** Believe that you have worked for the good fortune instead of looking at it as luck.
✓ **Business:** Set your business objectives concisely and build the business in your Mind Machine first.
✓ **Energy:** Imagine vast amounts of magnetic energy attaching to your body for the use of helping yourself and others.

> **"We always think in pictures, so always Imagine your mental pictures as moving pictures not still pictures"**

3 Steps to More Attraction Power

1. Never make a negative statement on what you are looking to attract

2. Condition your mind daily to attract that which you want

3. Fall asleep at night by giving your subconscious directions to get what you want.

Affirmation: "Wealth, Prosperity, Success, Love is Mine Now!"

Thought Control

- You have complete control over your thoughts
- What ever you think about will manifest unless you neutralize it by a contrary thought.
- Your sub-conscious mind moves as it is acted upon by your thoughts

Exercise- The Mental Attraction Bank

1. Envision a great bank

2. You have the key to all that is in there.

3. You can withdraw or add deposits when you want

4. You can transfer to others

"GOD IS IN CONTROL SO BE NOT AFRAID".
"GOD IS YOUR EMPLOYER"

Exercise- Attraction Imagination Exercise

1. Imagine the local bank mgr/ woman/man of choice/ job of choice/ vacation/ anything you want coming up to you and congratulating you on a job well done.

2. In your imagination hear a friend saying....

   a. What a bank account he/she has

b. What a beautiful wife or handsome husband

c. He/she has the best job

d. Can you imagine going to where he/she goes on Vacation?

3. I am attracting to me _____ because I am ethical, moral and looking to help my fellow man in all I do

Exercise- In your Mind, Think of Attracting

- ✓ Harmony
- ✓ Success
- ✓ Prosperity

Increase the Power of Your Mind > Plant in your mind the following:

1. Thought

2. Feeling

3. Imagination

Targeting Your Objectives with Authority

- **Goals must be Written, Dated and reviewed daily:** The key to achieving your objectives is to not only have the goals written down, but that you review them several times daily.
- **How to attract your goals like magic:** Use the Mind Machine as the mechanism with which to attract the objects of your desire. Use all of the principles of the mind and attraction and things will come to you in ways that seem
- **How to Goal Get not just Goal set:** Focus on the goal as being something that you have already achieved in the past. Once you already own the goal or objective in your mind, it will reveal itself into reality.
- **Why people miss their goals**-:Lack of Belief and faith in the obtaining the goal. Quitting before you should. Never back off of a goal, and if you miss it just reset it.
- **Goal Visualization:** Make it clear, concise and as real as you can. (see visualization sections)
- **Creating a probable future**: Believe in the possibilities and go after your goals and dreams with relentless determination.

Affirmation: "My words heal, quicken, vitalize, prosper, satisfy, persuade & make rich everyone I meet."

CHAPTER 6: Bonus Section: **Napoleon Hill's Success Principles**

Here are some of the principles have helped thousands of people to become wealthy in all areas of their life. Study these principles and put them into practice and you will surely know the meaning of getting out of life exactly what you want and expect.

The Power of the Mind- Napoleon Hills Principles

The Power of Definite Purpose*

- The starting point of all individual achievement is the adoption of a definite purpose and a definite plan for its attainment

- Any dominating idea, plan or purpose held in the mind, through repetition of thought, and emotionalized with a burning desire for its attainment, is taken over by the subconscious section of the mind and is acted upon, and it is thus carried through to its logical climax by whatever natural means may be available

- Any dominating desire, plan, or purpose held in the conscious mind and backed by absolute faith in its realization is taken over and acted upon by the subconscious section of the mind, and there is no known record of this kind of a desire having ever been without fulfillment.

- The power of thought is the only thing over which any person has complete, unquestionable control- a fact so astounding that it connotes a close relationship between the mind of man and the universal mind of infinite intelligence, and the connecting link between the two being Faith.

- The Subconscious portion of the mind is the doorway to Infinite Intelligence, and it responds to one's demands in exact proportion to the quality of one's Faith! The subconscious mind may be reached through faith and given instructions as though it were a person of a complete entity unto itself

- A definite purpose, backed by absolute faith is a form of wisdom, and wisdom in action produces positive results.

The Fundamentals of Faith: *

1) Definiteness of Purpose supported by personal initiative or action.

2) The habit of going the extra mile in all human relationships.

3) A Master Mind Alliance with one or more people who radiate courage based on Faith, and who are suited spiritually and mentally to ones needs in carrying out a given purpose.

4) A positive mind, free from all negatives, such as fear, envy, greed, hatred, jealousy and superstition. (A positive mental attitude is the first and most important of the Twelve Riches).

5) Recognition of the truth that every adversity carries with it the seed of an equivalent benefit; that temporary defeat is not failure until it has been accepted as such.

6) The habit of affirming one's Definite Major Purpose in life, in a ceremony of meditation, at least once daily.

7) Recognition of the Existence of Infinite Intelligence which gives orderliness to the universe; that all are minute expressions of this Intelligence, and as such the individual mind has no limitations except those which are accepted and setup by the individual in his own mind.

8) A careful inventory (in retrospect) of one's past defeats and adversities, which will reveal the truth that all such experiences carry the seed of an equal or greater benefit.

9) Self-respect expressed through harmony with one's own conscience.

10) Recognition of the oneness of all mankind.

* From The Master Key to Riches by Napoleon Hill

Mind Force Meditation: Mind Portal

By A. Thomas Perhacs

Published by Velocity Group Publishing

PO Box 9516 Hamilton, NJ 08650   www.advancedmindpower.com   www.mindforcesecrets.com

Introduction To Mind Portal

*Parts of this manuscript were previously included in my first work on meditation, entitled "Mastery Through Meditation"

From Mastery To Beyond

Mind Portal is a course designed to help you to take your meditation practices to the next level of proficiency. I have compiled the best concepts that I have learned over the years in meditation, remote sensing, viewing and other esoteric arts and have combined them with the *internal mind training* experience that I have learned from the internal chi arts from China and Japan.

When I write, I only keep the neccesary information. Why write 10 pages, when something can be summed up with one word? My goal is to provide to you an excellent system of meditation to increase your sensitivity to produce unique skills. Mind Portal does just that....

Meditation is a way for you get more control of your time and life. By investing a small amount of time per day, you will be paid back many times over from the benefits to your health, relationships, and a better understanding of how your body, mind and spirit work.

Meditation: "A devotional exercise to plan or intend in the mind, or to contemplate".

When many people think of meditation they visualize a swami or monk sitting cross-legged on a pillow in deep contemplation of what the meaning of life is. Although this is accurate, what we are teaching is how to use meditation to create a more compelling future for your life. This includes combining actual physical and mental exercises designed to trigger positive results within the brain.

This type of training is geared toward creating a habit of continually putting good information into your computer (brain) so that you can go towards anything that you want. This mental training will build a muscle (if you will) within your brain that will make you mentally strong, just as you could be physically strong from physical activity.

Chapter 1: Disciplining The Power & Creating Good Habits

Habits Determine Your Future

If You Change Your Habits, You Change Your Life, Forever

All success in life is based on habits. All problems or challenges that we have are based on (bad) habits. Habits are what we are, what we do, and why we do them.

Why do we eat too much?

Why do we smoke too much?

Why do we use too much bad language?

Why do we indulge in negative behavior such as drugs, alcohol, or other unhealthy lifestyle choices?

All things that we do, whether they are good or bad, are based on our habits.

Not all habits are bad, but virtually everything we do is based on habit: getting up for work; our workout routines (or lack thereof); our eating habits; our ability to be prepared for things; etceteras. Simply put: Everything we do is based on habit. Holding this maxim as true, it follows that…

"If you can control your habits you can control your life"

Discipline + Habits = Control

The only way you can really affect your habits is to create discipline. Well that sounds nice, but most people don't have any! Discipline is one of those dirty words, which most don't want to know.

Discipline can be learned and the most interesting thing is the way to become disciplined is to create a habit of discipline. You usually can't just jump into things, but what you can do is to break down the habit, so that it is bite sized, not huge for the person to do.

21 Days To Create a Habit

It only takes about 21 days to create a habit. That is why you see so many books that say learn _____ in 21 days. 21 days is the magic number if you will that you need to get through.

So if you need to lose 30 pounds in 3 months, it really is only 21 days from being accomplished. If you want to achieve **"Mind Portal"**, then you have only 21 days to get that under control.

In essence, the first 21 days or 3 weeks is the most important time when you are looking to create a new habit or looking to unload an old one. This is important information that you need to internalize.

21 days and you got it!

21 one days and you own it!

Whatever the habit is, 21 days and you are that habit.

Of course, realize that bad or destructive habits can be built in 21 days as well; it is therefore important that you are consciously focusing on the positive and not the negative.

Discipline The Power

When you can discipline yourself about anything, you become in total control of that activity. Discipline combined with habits gives you the foundation for long-term success. Discipline is the essence of what makes you successful. When you have discipline it is the thing that separates those that will pay whatever price their goals and dreams demand.

By linking discipline with your habits, you will have the ingredients that very few people have. How many people will discipline themselves to do the things that are necessary for their chosen skill, profession, sport or undertaking? Very few do; if you make the decision to just do a little more than the average, you will achieve more than the average.

If you can discipline yourself to do a daily meditation that allows you relax your body and take your mind to a higher level of understanding, you will have more than most people could even imagine. This is a simple thing, a 20-minute investment per day that can pay you in terms of large amounts of satisfaction in all areas of your life.

If it seem like we are repeating some things over, we are. We are trying to get the point across that success in life is as simple as listening daily to a pre-programmed meditation tape that is a step by step blueprint for your life, a meditation program that you can update at any time as your goals are met.

Controlling Your Destiny Through Meditation

When you create the habit of discipline, you are creating the control that is needed to reach your goals and objectives. The control is the meditation itself, which is a very simple way to direct yourself to your goals or any objectives that you want. It is enjoyable and will become something that you look forward to on a daily basis; it is not a task that you will dread and cause you to be unmotivated.

As you begin to relax your body and mind, you will truly realize that you control your life and that you are the captain of your own ship. As your mind expands and you get control of your body and mind, you will be able to reach into higher levels of your consciousness, giving you a much different perspective on life than ever before.

Programming The Mind For Success Through Meditation

The reason why meditation is so powerful in the process for success is that it is a controllable activity that requires little effort and can be duplicated by anyone. It does not require a specific ability or talent and can be learned very easily.

When you put your body in a meditative state, it is very similar to being in a **hypnotic trance.** When you are in a trance, the subliminal portion of the brain is more open to suggestions you introduce to it.

The key to any type of influencing to your brain, is you make the mind and body comfortable and relaxed enough that the concepts that you are introducing to it are accepted. Getting to a deeper state of relaxation allows your body and mind to relax, thus helping you to direct information and affirmations into the subliminal portion of the mind.

Understanding this, we are going to give you more techniques on how you can influence the mind.

In order to influence the mind you need to do the following on a consistent basis:

1. Get the body into a total state of relaxation;
2. Concentrate on going even deeper into that state;
3. Introduce the concepts of your goals and/or affirmations;
4. Visualize the outcomes of the goals with very specific mental images;
5. Always speak into existence- not what is, but what can be;
6. Always use the present tense for all affirmations. Example: I am a highly successful _____(fill in the blank for what you want);
7. Focus on these daily.

When the body is relaxed, your mind can better receive any instructions that you send to it. By getting the body into a deeper level of relaxation, you can deliver the instructions for your success in Life.

Everyone Is "Brain Washed"

"Brain washed" is really not a good word in most people's minds. However, anytime we are influenced in a very strong manner, and that influence sinks into our subconscious minds, it is a form of brain washing.

A better term would be **"brain influencing"**, in that you are being influenced by a certain group, person or doctrine.

The positive way to look at this is to realize that you have the ability to control what influences you. You can control all external and internal influences that you have in your life. Make the decision to decide how you are going to be influenced. You decide whom you associate with; you decide what television or movies you watch. Keep this in mind and you will realize that you always had the control of your life.

1. Television
2. Commercials & Advertisements
3. Our Parents, Colleagues, Companies

You Can Control Your Programming

By setting up a program that is specifically tailored by you for your own goals

and objectives, you will maintain a level comfort and control in your life that most people never have. The "true you" is what you believe to be true about yourself, whether it is "true" or not at the time. Through meditation, you can influence yourself to become the person that you want to be.

When programming a computer, it is the computer operator that controls the data which is put into the computer.

The types of input you introduce to your brain is totally up to you. If you put bad information into the computer, you will get bad information out of the computer. It is the old **"Reap what you sow"**.

The goal is to put in the things that are going to affect us in a positive way, not a negative one. This is a very central idea and is why affirmations and autosuggestion work so well.

Chapter 2: Meditative Postures & Control

Structure of Meditation

There are many different postures that you can use for your meditations. The most common posture is sitting cross-legged on the floor with a pillow.

Although this is what most people recognize as meditation, it may not be the right posture for everyone. The key is to be flexible and use what works best for YOU, not what someone else may dictate to you. Here are some postures and their advantages/disadvantages.

- **Lying Down**: This is the posture that we recommend to start with as it allows your body to relax the easiest. The downside in the beginning is that some people complain that they fall asleep when they lay down. You can correct this by teaching your body how to relax and refocus your mind for the meditation process instead of sleeping;
- **Sitting in a Chair:** This is recommended second to the lying down posture. You sit in a chair with your back straight, hands resting on your knees or lap. The chair is a good method to learn how to relax as we spend a lot of time sitting in chairs and you want to get to the point where you can relax your body at any time;
- **Sitting with legs crossed**: This is the vision of the swami or monk sitting cross-legged on a pillow. We only recommend this when you can sufficiently relax the body down by sitting in a chair or lying down. For most people, to sit this way for 20 minutes or more would be uncomfortable, but if you can truly relax in this position, by all means do so.
- **Standing**: This is primarily for energy development (See SPC-USA's Chi Power Training course) and is not an option within this course. When you stand, you are putting stress on the body. When you can stand for 20 minutes and relax the body in a stressful situation, you will gain a different kind of relaxation- the ability to relax while under stress.

Musical Considerations

If you meditate with music, make sure that it is something that is soothing and will put your mind and body in a relaxed state not a stressful or negative one. Music has a lot more power than most would think, so it is very important to select your meditation music wisely.

Using a light piano or natural sound usually works better than lyrics, since you will be making suggestions to your subconscious mind throughout the process.

43

Keeping Distractions To The Minimal

When meditating, it is important that you keep distractions to a minimum. If possible, isolate yourself from distractions. Some people like to get up early in the morning to do their meditation as they find fewer distractions at that time.

Other people like to do it at night before they go to sleep. Any time is fine. What you may want to do is experiment and see what time works best for you and your life's schedule.

Sometimes, depending on your situation, you may find that you need to go somewhere to do your meditation. Some people will go to a park or the beach to get away. This can be a good way to separate your self from the normal distractions of life, but also could prove harder to control.

The key to any meditation is to do it consistently. Find a place that you can do your meditation and keep it minimized with distractions.

Keeping The Bladder Empty

Keeping the bladder empty is a key to any type of meditation program. This is an important thing to keep in mind, but many have never been told. When the bladder is full, your body will not be able to relax as well as when it is empty. When the body is fully and completely relaxed, you will be able to better get the results for which you are looking.

Relaxed Belly Breathing

Relaxed belly breathing or chi breathing is when you focus your breathing within your stomach. Most people breathe more through their chest than through the belly. This is due to stress.

Babies always breathe through the efficiency of belly breathing, but as we get older and stress starts to take a hold of us, we start to move our breathing higher up into the chest. The key is to always do your breathing in a relaxed manner.

When you inhale your stomach should go out slightly and when you exhale the belly should go in. This is Chi Breathing or relaxed belly breathing.

Meditation Clothes

Your body puts of an energy wave called Chi. Every culture has an understanding of this kind of energy, but with different names. The basic understanding is that we are essentially beings comprised of [bio-electromagnetic] energy.

As you do your meditation sessions, you are going to create an aura of the person that you want to be. By doing this it will positively affect all areas of your life. This includes the clothes that you wear while you are training.

The best types of clothes to wear are clothes that are natural fibers, such as 100% cotton. When you wear the same clothes during your sessions, the positive energy that you are putting off will actually attach itself to the clothes.

After a time they will become "chi clothes". You will also notice the energy of the room as well as the chair or bed that you are using in your training to have a specific energy feel to it as well.

Visualizing What You Desire

Anytime you are meditating, you want to use positive visualization of the things that you want to achieve. When you can visual something, you can get the mental picture that you will need in order to turn your goals and dreams into realities.

Visualizing what you want is very powerful; when combined with autosuggestion and affirmations, it is a super charged method of helping you to reach your goals and objectives.

When you can see, through your mind's eye, the exact thing that you want to accomplish, you will start to manifest that in the physical world. **This may take a little while to get under your control, as you will have to practice daily to get the techniques of relaxation down to create the mental results you are trying to achieve.** That is the importance of including affirmations and visualization in your daily meditations.

we want and to get rid of those we don't. You will be able to focus better on several areas at once due to the powerful affirmations that you will use to reach your objectives. You can set these affirmations for any area of your life, such as:

- Getting in Shape or Losing Weight;
- Working out Regularly;
- Maintaining Focus
- Personal/Business Goals

The Structure of Meditation

The structure of the meditation is very important. You must have a format to follow in the beginning so that your body can relax; this will aid you in trusting yourself to go even deeper into the meditative state. You will receive in depth instructions on how you can get to the meditative state.

The following are good guidelines to follow when putting together a personalized meditation session. The concepts are standard, but the words should be your own, so that you will talk to yourself in your normal tones and inflections. The outline also gives several options, so see which ones you like and implement them into your meditation program.

1. **Relax the body down (always concentrate on making arms, legs and eyes heavy):**

   - Each body part at a time (toes, arch, ankles, calf, knees, etc) causing them to start to feel heavy;
   - General Message- "My legs are getting heavy, my arms are getting heavy", etc.;
   - Your Total body- "My entire body is going into a complete state of relaxation".

2. **Breathe Deeply from the belly:**

   - Take in a deep breath and hold it; exhale slowly, releasing all anxieties, problems and concerns;
   - Relax your body deeper with each exhale.

3. **Count down from 10 to 1:**

   - Relaxing the body even deeper on each count;
   - Sometimes go from 25 to 1 or for shorter times 3 to 1.

4. **Feel the body relax & get heavy, like floating on a cloud:**

   - Feel the body getting warmer and more comfortable;
   - "My body is getting so relaxed that I can no longer feel it".

5. **Keeping telling your body to relax deeper and deeper:**

   - "My mind is at ease, my thoughts do not wander; I am more and more relaxed."

6. **Picture yourself going deeper into yourself:**

   - Your body falling;
   - Your body rising;
   - Experiment with both.

7. **Affirmations & specific instructions of what you want (choose and create affirmations that are specific to you):**

   - I am relaxed and in control at all times;
   - I am bold and confident;
   - I am in the process of becoming the person I desire to be.
   - I am a positive influence on everyone I come in contact with.

8. **Different Modes that you can do while meditating:**

   - Visualization of Goals (actual visualizing them as being real and already happening);

- Go to a specific place in your mind to relax you more (the beach, the woods, space);
- A private workshop within your mind to work out challenges or situations you are facing;
- Total Blank (Thinking about nothing- Mind is blank);
- Healing a specific ailment that you or a loved one has.

9. **Give final instruction when you emerge from the meditation:**

- I will feel refreshed as if sleeping for several hours;
- I will focus more strongly on affirmations;
- I will succeed and have a successful day - "I believe in the perfect outcome of every situation in my life".

The key to this entire process is getting the body to relax down as much as possible. Keep telling your body to "relax down". Sometimes you may need to speak to each body part several times until it begins to relax down. Relaxation is what is going to give you the results that you want.

Chapter 3: Going Deeper Into Meditation

Meditate for 20-30 Minutes Per Day

You must build up the habit of doing your meditations for a minimum of 20 minutes per day. These 20 minutes will start to be a focal point to the beginning of your day or the completion of your day. Of course, as you get into the practice of doing your meditation, you can increase it to 30 minutes per session or you can do two sessions per day. Some people may even get up to an hour of meditation per day based on their needs and acceptance of the practice.

As you start to follow through on this new habit, you will soon discover that this habit is transferable to other areas of your life. The key to creating success in life is to make a habit of the things we want and to get rid of those we don't. You will be able to focus better on several areas at once due to the powerful affirmations that you will use to reach your objectives. You can set these affirmations for any area of your life, such as:

- Getting in Shape or Losing Weight;
- Working out Regularly;
- Maintaining Focus

Strength of Concentration- Getting Into a Trance Like State

The idea of increasing the strength of your concentration is vital for this process to work. When your strength of concentration is focused, you begin to enter into a "trance like" state, where you can manipulate what you are trying to achieve.

When we can get to this trance like state, we start to access the higher portions of our brain, giving deeper access to the subliminal portion of the mind. This allows you get your affirmations deeply imbedded into your being.

You put yourself in a trance like state every time you watch TV, or drive a car. Trance like states are akin to these almost automatic responses.

The reason advertisers put subliminal messages on TV or magazine ads are to influence your deeper mind. If advertisers can do this (and they don't even know you), think how much more effective you can be if you program your mind to lead you to the things in life that you want?

You can increase your strength of concentration by also doing the following:

- Gazing at a candle;
- Staring at hypnotic charts (which we can supply);
- Focusing on a single object;
- Putting your mind towards a "Singleness of Purpose".

Chapter 4: Spiritual Travel

Third Eye Focusing

Many people that study meditative practices become aware of the 3rd Eye or Pineal Gland that is within the inside of the head. The 3rd eye is the area between your eyebrows and is considered the psychic center of your body. The penal gland is situated behind the 3rd eye, closer to the middle of the inside of your skull.

Being that this is a psychic center, the 3rd eye can be activated through your meditative practices. The key to opening up this center is to get your body to totally relax down and get into a deep state of meditation.

The functioning of the 3rd eye is responsible for greater levels of knowledge and spiritual understanding. Although some may open the 3rd eye in a relatively short amount of time, it may take others years to get this under control. With this type of knowledge comes the responsibility that accompanies all gifts and talents.

To open this area up, start to view the 3rd eye while you are doing your meditation. Again this can take a long period of time, so be patient and learn to relax down.

Just remember that your 3rd eye will open when you least expect it and also while you are not really trying. Some practitioners have been known to experience strange side effects and experiences when the 3rd eye opens.

Exercise: Focusing on the 3rd Eye Opening

Step #1: Get into a relaxed meditative position

Step #2: Use relaxation methods to calm the body down

Step #3: Still the mind by deep breathing

Step #4: With the mind stilled and the body relaxed start to view the area between your eyebrows, the 3rd eye

Step #5: Stay focused on that point and maintain the relaxation

Out of Body Experiences & Lucid Dreaming

As you get deeper into meditation, you may start to experience many different strange feelings and occurrences. This could be a thing such as Out of Body Experiences (OBE), déjà vu (recognizing a place or situation that you have never experienced before) and Lucid Dreaming (where the dream is very realistic and you are in total control).

Once you realize that during your sleep, your spirit will generally leave your body, a lot of these things won't seem as strange. We really are spiritual beings living in a shell called our body. Our body is really carrying around our spirit and is no more significant than your car getting you from point A to point B. Every religion or religious experience recognizes this fact and you can find a plethora of information backing up these concepts.

The OBE is when you have full recognition of the spirit leaving the body and going somewhere else. Many that have done this have traveled to a friend's house, another country or another world. Again, your spirit can travel anywhere that your mind can see it traveling to.

Some think that this goes against some religious doctrine, but in reality, it actually confirms a lot (if not all) of religious doctrine from: Christianity; Judaism; Islam; Hinduism; and other religions of the world. Don't fear; remember that God is in control at all times.

When you lucid dream, you are actually controlling the circumstances of the dream sequence. From my experience, I feel the Lucid Dream is more of an OBE, that you remember as a dream. In most cases, you will wake up and have a very vivid remembrance of a dream. This dream however will feel more like a memory of an experience rather than a random dream.

One key to remembering Lucid Dreams or experiences is to focus on your hands. If you can visually see your hands while in this dream state, you can actually control the action taking place in this state.

Also keep in mind, when in the dream state, your body is not bound by the limitations of the physical world, so condition yourself to experience some of the following:

- Walking Through Walls

- Flying

- Breathing Under Water

- Travelling Through Space

- Being Invisible

When you condition your mind to create and produce these types of scenarios, it will respond by helping you to experience concepts that while inside of your physical body seem impossible.

50

Astral Projection

Some Keys to Getting Your Spirit Out

- The ability to relax your body 100% and stay lucid.
- You have to shift your consciousness to a point outside of your physical body.

- Build up and control your mental energy & chi to relax into the projection without either falling asleep or allowing the spirit to pop back into the body.

Some Unique Ways to Get Outside of Your Body

- Imagine yourself climbing a ladder or rope
- Imagine yourself as a point of light floating on top of water in a rapidly filling tank. Your task is to exit through a tiny hole in the roof of the tank
- Imagine a mirror image of yourself twenty to thirty feet behind you. See yourself moving backwards towards it.
- Start by imagining your energy hands being able to lift out of your body and pull and move your chi to your legs and other parts of your body.
- See a mirror image of yourself in front of you and slowly merge towards it.
- Breath through the pores of your body until there is no more recognition of the physical body.
- While sitting in a chair, imagine a horizontal bar above your line of sight. Push yourself to see over it with your spirit body only. Hold your breath in when you get a sensation of rising.
- Tighten the muscles in your feet and hands, then contract your entire body and see yourself falling in your minds eye (3rd eye)
- Feel yourself being in a whirlpool of energy moving clockwise. Feel yourself being sucked down through the vortex of the whirlpool. Feel the sensations of contraction then expansion of the spirit body.
- Imagine being taken and carried on the crest of a big wave (like a surfer).
- See and feel a point of light energy a couple of feet in front of you. Feel it slowly approach. When it reaches you, blend in with the and become part of the light energy.
- In a sitting posture, see a mirror image of yourself directly in front of you. Repeat your name over and over until it becomes almost unrecognizable. Then imagine, feel and see the person as the real you.
- Focus on the 3rd eye and feel the vibration after a while. See the darkness.
- Then see the little speck of light through the darkness and go towards it. As you get closer to the light, the darkness will fade and you can exit the body.
- Focus your body as a full and complete energy body. As it begins to resonate higher, begin to feel your spirit start to step out, pull out or jump out of your physical shell (body).

Keep in mind that you will need to try each of these techniques to see which ones will work best for you. No one can determine which ones will work best for you.

Each of these techniques contains a method that absolutely works. Apply these methods with the meditation CD/MP3 that comes with the Mind Portal course, and you will have a very good set of strategies to enable you to get these concepts to work for you.

Themes For Travelling

These mental training methods are very valuable in order to get the body relaxed and accepting of getting the mind to be aware of feelings outside of the body from a spiritual sense. Use each one and see which one is the easiest for your body and mind to adapt to. You mind find several combined work as well.

1. Floating
2. Rising up and down
3. Sinking
4. Space, woods, beach
5. Stepping out of the body
6. Climbing out with a ladder or rope

Chapter 5: Remote Sensing, Viewing & Influencing

Tapping Into Your Subconscious Mind

The process of producing information that accurately describes a person, place, event or object while being in a totally different place, is referred to as "Remote Viewing".

As you become more aware and comfortable with your body and mind, you will start to be able to control the energies and new sensations within your body and mind. One of the most unique skills is to be able to sense things remotely by tapping into the powers of your subconscious mind.

How this differs from actually releasing the spirit as in an OBE or Astral Travel, Remote Viewing does not require you leaving your body (although many Remote Viewers do).

Remote Viewing or Sensing is more along the lines of you seeing into your Third Eye like it is a computer or TV monitor and you are extracting information via this method.

The subconscious knows everything that you have done and everything that you will know or do! This is an interesting concept, but unfortunately most people will never harness the ability to tap into it.

By consistently doing your meditation, you can gain the ability to tap into that reservoir of knowledge. Remote sensing is how you can sense things at a distance. By relaxing down you can start to pick things up at a distance.

Maybe start out by just seeing into the next room and then expanding from there. You can also start to feel things in the room without even touching them. Again, like everything we are doing here, it is a process and may work right away for some while others may require years to develop these skills. You can do anything that your mind can conceive.

Remote influencing is the idea that you can influence someone from a distance. By focusing your mental powers, you can send energy out to influence people in a positive way or to help them overcome sickness or problems.

Again, the mind is your link to doing all of these things. Sometimes when you do these things, the subjects will even feel your presence. Have you ever picked up the phone, knowing who was on the other line? That is the subconscious giving you a glimpse of what can be.

Remote Viewing Projects

Once you learn how to tap into the subconscious part of the mind and begin the process of remote viewing, you will be able to accurately predict certain occurances. Such as the following

1. Describe people, places and things
2. Produce informational leads
3. Reconstruct events
4. Decision making made easier
5. Making predictions

Some Keys To Remote Viewing

When looking to Remote View or any types of Advanced Meditative Practices, the key is to relax and don't make things too complicated. The more complicated and involved you make things, the more of a chance you will not get them to work.

- Having your own protocol
- Physical relaxation & focus
- Centering yourself and stilling the mind
- Slowing down body responses
- Reducing Sensory input and processes
- Increased awareness of internal processes such as dreams and fantasy. Knowing the difference between imagination and reality
- Centering yourself and stilling the mind
- Realization that time is an illusion

Remote Viewing With a Partner

Many of the top Remote Viewers conduct their remote viewing sessions with a partner, who acts as a control for the information on where the Remote Viewing is taking place.

There are several different ways to look at this and I will do my best to describe them to you.

The first aspect, is when a partner has a project target in a closed envelope for you to locate. This target can be anything. It can be a person, place or thing. It could even be something in the room you are in.

The partner will let you know if it is a person, place or thing so that you can start to narrow down what it is you are viewing. This will take a lot of concentration and practice to become proficient at this.

The second aspect of this would be where you know exactly where you are going. You are using the partner to allow you to stay focused on what you are viewing. In my experience, it is good to use a partner as well as conduct solo target practice, so you can learn by yourself.

Anytime you can get a partner involved, you will be able to have a higher rate of succes. Many times, you can even get a partner involved in the OBE and Astral Projection methods as well.

Practice Every Day

Remote Viewing, like any developed skill takes a lot of "Flight Time". Some are natural Remote Viewers, but most of us come to this type of training without a natural ability.

The best way to get these concepts to work, is to devote 30 minutes or more per day working on specific techniques. Do not get discouraged because your mind relys on your belief factor in order to get these types of powerful techniques to work for you...

If everyone was able to do this, it would not be such a special talent, wouldn't you agree?

When I was actively pursuing my training in OBE's and Remote Viewing, I often times practiced several times per day, at different times of the day, to try and catch my body when it could get to the right state of relaxation.

In some cases, I would begin meditating at 12 midnight and see if I could get out then, while still being lucid. Sometimes I fell asleep, other times I achieved an outcome I was looking for.

More Important Keys

Stay focused on your training and look at this like any other type of training you are doing for a predescribed outcome.

1. Don't get disapointed if it doesn't happen immediately

2. Talk to your body to keep relaxing down more (this is a form of self hypnosis)

3. Vary your training and use different methods and techniques

4. Don't always expect something to happen- Just relax (In the beginning, you will get out more when you least expet it than when you do.)

Chapter 6 Creating Personal Magnetism

Creating Magnetism With Your Energy

You can create a magnetism that will attract others to you by harnessing the energy that you put off; send this bio- electromagnetic energy out in a pattern that will cause everyone you meet to want to know you.

Have you ever seen someone with a very magnetic personality? They don't necessarily have to look attractive either; they just have to have that quality that makes people want to be around them.

When you make people feel good when they are around you, you will create a synergistic effect for all around you. Always keep a positive attitude.

Always compliment people when you meet them. Always have something good to say.

When you act this way, you instantly separate yourself from 95% of most people out there. Most people are attracted to people who treat them nice, with respect and are generally interested in them as people.

Be the type of person that lifts people up and you will notice that you will always have a personal magnetism that will attract others to you.

Creating a personal magnetism could take a little while, but like everything else in this course you, must work on it. Be objective about your weaknesses and then work on them. The more you can find the flaws in your personality or how you deal with people, the more you will get an understanding of how you can attract others to you.

Once you can attract people to you, then you can start to influence people. Remember that there are three reasons why people will be attracted to you and will be influenced by you: Knowledge; Affection; Trust.

- ✓ **They Know You:** As you get to know people, you will become more of an influence in their life;
- ✓ **They Like You:** When people like you, they will begin to be more and more influenced by you based on your past experiences with them;
- ✓ **They Trust You:** People will begin to trust you based on the reliable persona that you give. As such, you will influence them more.

When you meet people, you should allow them the opportunity to get to know you by sharing things about your life to which they will relate. As you relate personal information to them, they will then realize that you are very much like them, and as such, they will start to trust you.

Once people feel like they know you and like you, they will start to trust you. These are three important things to remember as you are working on your personal magnetic power over people.

Creating Voice Energy & Power

Your voice is a powerful tool that you can use for the benefit of others. You can build up an energy voice that will project more than just the words that you say...

Your voice alone can project any other emotion or concept that you want to reveal to a person.

The different types of tones that you use on someone determine a large part the reaction you get from the person. If you are angry and yell at someone, what kind of result can you expect back?

Just by changing the tone of your voice you can control situations. If someone is angry with you, lower your voice and speak very softly.

This will make their anger subside, as people can only be angry with someone who is being angry back with them. By changing the tone of your voice you can then control the conversation.

By deepening your voice and speaking from far back in your throat, you will cause a great amount of energy to come forth with your words. Your words should be spoken very measured and precise to get the desired results.

The more precise and confident that you are will determine your results of what you are trying to get across to your subject.

When you speak bold and confidently and add a powerful energy to it, people will naturally listen to you more as they will feel the energy that you project.

Be careful with your power voice, as it could contain too much energy, if you use it in an uncontrolled fashion.

This is why you should only speak with words that encourage or make people feel good. We all may sometimes use an expletive, but this should be an exception not the rule of how you speak.

How you speak and the words you use let people know the type of individual you are. Use language and the power of chi wisely.

Chapter 7: Self Image Programming

This should be done into your computer or a tape recorder so you can hear the strength and power of your own voice. Remember that you can use the following meditations with your own affirmations and goals. You can also use any type of visualzation that you like as well. You may also focus on your third eye or work on your remote sensing and out of body skills as well.

Relax Down #1

"I am lying down, eyes closed, relaxed...My arms and legs are flexible...I am quite relaxed... Nothing can distract me... I am quite calm... I let myself be drawn along. I am breathing slowly, regularly... I am feeling quite well... A pleasant peacefulness envelops my body"

" I will take a deep breath and while exhaling will exhale all tension, stress and negativity in my life. It wil go away and I will feel refreshed and energized.

"Now, I am concentrating on my facial muscles... My cheek muscles are growing heavy, totally relaxed. My jaw muscles are totally relaxing down.... I am relaxing the muscles in my forehead and they are getting quite heavy... My entire facial area is relaxing down. My eyelids are heavy... Heavier and heavier... My eyes are hermetically closed... I can no longer open them... I no longer want to... My neck muscles are now relaxing down, I feel a comfort and relaxation throughout my head and neck.... Now I am concentrating on my torso, including my chest, back, stomach and all of my internal organs. These areas are now relaxing down.. ... My entire torso is relaxed... Feels heavy as if being drawn downward.... My arms are growing heavy... They are drawn downward... This heaviness prevades my arms more and more... More and more... Now, my arms are as heavy as lead. I am concentrating on my legs... I am quite calm... I clearly feel them growing heavy... More and more.... Now, my legs are quite heavy. As heavy as lead. I let myself sink more and more into this wonderful feeling of relaxation and heaviness... I am more and more relaxed... More and more relaxed"

"With each exhale my body goes deeper and deeper into this state of relaxation and heaviness. I will now teach my body to relax down even more.... I will countdown from 3-1 and I will get more relaxed with each count... I will go deeper with each count.

3.........I am going ten times deeper than the moment before;

2........ I am going twenty times deeper than the moment before;

1........ I am going one hundred times deeper than the moment before.

"Nothing can distract me... I hear only my voice... I feel myself sinking still more, more and more deeply into this feeling of peace... I feel quite well... I am sinking deeper and deeper... More and more."

"Every cell, in every part of my body, has now risen to a higher state of power... Is glowing like a high-energy dynamo... Is giving off magnetism and chi that turns others irresistibly towards me... That pulls what I want and what I need out of my surroundings.

"My body is now surrounded by this invisible field of physical magnetism and chi... It never tires... It never dims... It is always there to protect me... To draw to me what I want... I have the self-confidence I have always dreamed of... I can now make my dreams become my realities... I have the power to do this because God has blessed me with this power..."

- *I have total faith and belief in my ability to control all areas in my life, based on the power with which God has blessed me;*

- *I am disciplined & stay focused on my goals;*

- *I am relaxed and in control at all times;*

- *I am a positive influence on everyone with whom I come in contact;*

- *I expect success every day;*

- *I am bold and confident;*

- *I keep my thoughts pure and good, and channel my energy into creative, worthwhile actions;*

- *My mind is strong and I achieve all of my goals and objectives on time.*

"I will use this power wisely... It will help others at the same time it helps me... I will do no harm with it... It is too great to misuse... I will employ it for good only... For my good... and for the good of the world...

" When I come out of this state of relaxation I will feel as if I have been sleeping for several hours, fully refreshed and ready to take on any challenges and activities that the day holds."

Relax Down #2

" Now I will gently begin to relax my body. I will breathe as if deep sleeping. I am lying down, relaxing my body down. My stomach extends with each inhalling breath. I relax deeper on each exhale. I will concentrate my thoughts. I mentally visualize each muscle as it relaxes.

I breath through my belly in a slow relaxed breathing rhythm. Do not force the breath. Breath to continually feel my belly, rythmically, as if sleeping. Each muscle will now learn to relax".

"Now, relax the big toe of my left foot. Speak to it if necessary. Relax the big toe of the right foot. Go deeper with each exhale. Left toes, relax. Right toes relax. Left arch, relax. Right arch, relax. Left heel, relax. Right heel, relax. Go deeper with each exhale. Left ankle, relax. Right ankle, relax. Left calf, relax. Right calf, relax. Go deeper with each exhale".

"Remember to speak out loud to any part that does not cooperate. Left knee, relax. Right knee, relax. Left thigh, relax. Right thigh, relax. Buttocks, relax. Abdominal muscles, relax. Lower back, relax. Upper back, relax. Chest, relax. Go deeper with each exhale and speak to any part that does not stay relaxed.".

" Neck, relax. Cheeks, relax. Left eye, relax. Right eye, relax. Entire head, relax. Left shoulder, relax. Right shoulder, relax. Left upper arm, relax. Right upper arm, relax. Left elbow, relax. Right elbow, relax Go deeper with each exhale. Left forearm relax. Right Forearm, relax. Left wrist, relax. Right wrist, relax. Left hand, relax. Right hand, relax. Left fingers, relax. Right finger, relax. Left thumb, relax. Right thumb, relax. My entire body should now be competely relaxed. Remember to speak to any part which may have tensed again".

"My total body is relaxed; with each exhale I go deeper. I will now concentrate on the goals and objectives that I want to achieve. I will focus on the positive results that I

want to achieve in all areas of my life. When I am done with this, I will awaken from this state and feel refreshed, as though I have been sleeping for several hours.""

Creating Your Own Meditations

I have layed out the basic concepts and methods for the meditations, but keep in mind, you can modify them at any time using any of the pieces to customize it to fit your specific and individual needs. This is the uniquesness of this. These two relax down sessions are guidelines only and act as a way for you to begin the process...

Chapter 8: Final Considerations

Your Journey of a Lifetime Begins Here

Take the wonderful concepts you have learned in this manuscript and use them. Knowledge that is learned and is not used is a waste...

Once you begin to see the value these techniques will provide you will become very excited to the outcomes you will be able to achieve.

Stay focused and be persistant and you will be able to get these concepts to work for you.

It took me many years to hone down the knoweldge and skills contained in here, so keep doing the meditations daily to create a habit of success.

The exercises and meditations were specifically structured to enable you to get results quickly as long as you do them.

I wish you the best of luck and drop me a line and let me know how you like this.

Respectfully,

A. Thomas Perhacs

Updated Edition

August 2008

Mind Force Psychic Energy: Internal Power Centers

By A. Thomas Perhacs

Published by Velocity Group Publishing

PO Box 9516 Hamilton, NJ 08650 www.advancedmindpower.com www.mindforcesecrets.com

Chapter 1: MASTERING THE ENERGY OF BODY & MIND

The Conscious mind

The conscious mind is the ordinary everyday mind that we are all familiar with. It is born with the body and inevitably passes away with the body. During our lives, it analyzes and records all of our life experiences. Forming its myriad opinions about those experiences, it presents them to us as fact and has us believing that both the world around us and ourselves really are what it says we are.

The problem is that the information that the conscious mind receives through our five sense faculties and subsequently processes is often insubstantial and illusory, and so, based on those illusions, offers us not only an incomplete view of the world and ourselves, but creates for each of us our own very personal earthly heavens and hells, as well.

Unlike the subconscious mind, which is endowed with much greater capabilities and is operational continuously throughout all of our many incarnations, the conscious mind is limited by having to experience life anew each and every time we reincarnate. That is, at conception, it starts off blank like a brand new recording tape with nothing on it from our past to give us at least some semblance of a head start in life.

In a way, it is very much like the intellectual labors of Sisyphus where, instead of having to roll a large, cumbersome, stone up a steep seemingly unassailable hill, only to have it roll down again when it nears the top, we are rolling all of our conscious mind experiences up a hill only to have them suddenly disappear and reappear at the bottom, blank and inexperienced once again.

Through the offices of the conscious mind, reality is variously and personally distorted, subtly paving over much of the common ground that would otherwise unite us all in a singular experience of reality. Through the agency of the conscious mind, higher truths become subjective truths. That is, it forms concepts of reality that have their genesis in the arbitrary and self-serving interests of each individual conscious mind and therefore must be considered suspect, at best.

In analyzing the world and itself, it is here that the conscious mind ignorantly genuflects before the altar of truth that it, itself, has designed and constructed, and then in bewilderment, wonders why there are no answers flowing from that altar which will satisfy its seemingly unquenchable thirst not only for mundane answers, but for authentic spiritual knowledge, as well.

The arbitrary, individualistic, unreliable nature of the lower mind is exhibited quite often when two or more people view the same incident, and results in different interpretations of that event. It is the individual conscious mind's arbitrary interpretations of people, places, things, and events, that cloud the fundamental truth of their nature and, as a result, is responsible for the creation of so many of the spiritual and day-to-day misunderstandings and problems that we are plagued with. For this reason, wisdom in deciphering the true nature of existence is not, nor can it ever be, the conscious mind's forte.

All of this becomes even more understandable when we realize that the conscious mind bases all of its interpretations about the world on data that it receives from what are arguably inferior sense organs. When we compare our human experience of the world with that of the rest of the animal kingdom, for example, we seem to fall quite short. Consider a dog's sense of smell and hearing, for instance.

Here, we find that a dog's world is rife with odors and sounds that we are completely oblivious to. A shark's sense of smell is so acute that it can detect blood in water, one part in a million. To us the blood would be non-existent. What about of sense of sight? A hawk can spot a mouse stirring a field of wheat a mile away. At that distance, for us the mouse would not exist.

So it is with all of our senses - sight, hearing, touch, taste, and smell. Yet, our conscious mind takes the inferior information it receives and arbitrarily determines the nature of both the world and of us, as well. Still, such as it is, the sensory information that the conscious mind receives is all that it has to work with. Because of that, it denies those who rely on it the ability to pierce the veil of illusion that shields the truth of existence.

In fact, many of us because of our reliance on our conscious minds do not even recognize that the veil exists at all. Understand that when the eye first perceives an object, it does so quite pristinely, without the least vestige of prejudice. That is, it receives the image of the object without any preconceived ideas concerning it. The eye is simply seeing the object based on its particular physical ability, without labels, descriptive colorings, past memory correlations, or personal biases.

However, once the eye passes that image on to the conscious mind for interpretation, the object becomes variously distorted because the conscious mind then takes that image and superimposes on it all manner of correlative information, such as any past experiences it has on record concerning it or similar objects. Now, when it comes to our psychic abilities, the fact is that the conscious mind simply does not possess such capabilities.

Are you surprised?

This, of course, is not to say that the lower mind is not privy to such information. It is just that it does not receive psychic information through any innate psychic devices of its own. Instead, such information comes to it through the auspices and psychic faculties of the subconscious mind. Still, even through this process, the conscious mind falls short and is found sorely wanting.

The reason for this is that the conscious mind is often too loud and loquacious to hear, much less understand, the psychic information delivered to by the higher mind. Even when, during those rare moments when it is quiet enough to acknowledge the subconscious mind's psychic information, it immediately begins a subtle process of superimposing on that information a plethora of arbitrary distortions.

For this reason alone, it is imperative that those of us wanting to begin the process of mastery over our inner powers should not conduct that quest within the truth-distorting arena of the lower mind. Instead, you must learn how to quiet your conscious mind to the point where it is so reticent and unimposing that the higher mind with its wonderful psychic information gathering and transmitting capabilities come forward and dominate.

The Subconscious Mind

You can think of the subconscious mind as the unique and subtle part of us that has existed since our very first incarnation and serves to merge within us, both the temporal and the eternal; that of the

65

dark, gross, limited, physical world of the conscious mind and that of the pristine, limitless, eternal realm of our souls.

Since the subconscious mind is devoid of the reasoning faculties inherent in the conscious mind, it does not possess the ability to create the innumerable arbitrary distortions that reasoning processes often promote to obscure our vision of the world.

Even so, it should not be understood to mean that the subconscious mind is by any means perfect, it is not. The reason for this is that, like the conscious mind, the subconscious mind has also been recording our life's experiences, not just in our present life, but also from the very moment in our dim and distant pasts when we had first become a living entity, a sentient being.

What is more, it has not only been recording throughout all of our innumerous earthly incarnations but throughout all of our heaven and hell experiences in between those periods.

It is all recorded there and, under the proper conditions, can be made accessible to us. While receiving psychic information, the subconscious mind sometimes draws on its wealth of recorded experiences and finds correlative data there, data that it subsequently uses to bring that psychically received information into sharper focus, one that makes it somehow more identifiable.

The remainder of the time, however, the subconscious mind seems not to be so helpful and instead of making that psychically received information clearer, it actually produces the opposite effect, and obscures that data by superimposing on it what it thinks to be relevant correlative experiences.

Does that make the psychic information it receives invalid?

No, it doesn't mean that at all. On those occasions it simply places us in the position of having to peek under the veil it created in order to uncover the truth of the communication. That, in the final analysis, is really not so bad, is it?

Based on our research, it seems that we can consider the subconscious mind to actually be a subtle intermediary device created by the soul in order to connect it to the exterior world or world of matter.

In other words, the higher mind seems to be the link between the ephemeral outside of us and the glorious eternal inside of us. It is, therefore, the penultimate tool for the performance of supra-sensory perception and the application of supra-sensory principles and techniques.

We say penultimate, because the ultimate source of knowledge, wisdom, and power, of course, has to be the soul, itself. Since the subconscious mind seems to be such an easily accessible translator of the infinite amount of information contained within the soul's limitless precincts, it only seems reasonable that we who are seeking to understand the nature of our existence should make good use of it.

In short then, we would not be wrong in thinking of the subconscious mind as the golden key that will help us unlock the vast spiritual inner powers lying predominantly dormant within us.

The Soul

The soul is our true essence….

It is that part of the Eternal that has been locked inside the world of matter since the time of the creation and is the solitary, motivating, spiritual force that has been, not only responsible for giving rise to us and all other sentient life forms, but it is also the great mystical power deep within us that drives us ever onward in a deliberately linear spiritual evolution that will, in time, eventuate in our deliverance, our long awaited piece of personal salvation.

Our souls, being one with the Eternal, are the supreme sources of knowledge and wisdom where nothing is hidden and nothing is lacking. Within its pristine climes are the great mystical founts of divine potency that compel us to endure the incessant changes of life in our efforts to rise above the illusions of the world and to deliberately seek after that which is enduring and of true value, to seek the eternal.

To this end, we must understand that our souls are the definitive reality, the ultimate pot of gold at the end of our personal spiritual rainbows. Our souls, being the divine presence of God within us, are the ultimate mystical gateways that will lead us out of this world of pain and suffering.

Through its portals, each of us must pass if our personal cycles of reincarnation are to come to an end and we are to return to our spiritual home, finally shed of the impediments that have kept us away so long.

Our souls have not only provided us with a wonderful variety of psychic tools with which to explore and understand ourselves and the truths concerning the matrix of existence, but, more importantly, they have given us the means with which to fulfill our personal evolutionary and spiritual destinies. All that we have to do is to take advantage of its infinite bounty.

Chi (Energy)

Throughout this study, we will see the term "Chi" used frequently. Chi comes from Sanskrit, the ancient language of India, and means "life force" or "life energy." It is the energy that not only sustains us in life, but sustains all of creation, as well. It is the primal, indivisible, indigo-colored, energy of manifest existence, without which nothing could exist.

Chi has been called by other names: ki, chi, m'retz na'she... the terms are really quite interchangeable. When we consider the role Chi plays in our psychic abilities, it is evident that no such abilities could exist or function without it.

The rule is: The more Chi we have available for use, the greater, and more substantial our psychic potentials are.

Why?

For the simple reason that during episodes of telepathy, clairvoyance, psychometry, etc., we have come to understand that Chi functions in the capacity of a carrier wave, similar to the carrier waves so necessary for radio transmission.

That is, just as a carrier wave in radio broadcasting is originally pure and un-modulated (carrying no information), similarly, a stream of projected Chi is pure and un-modulated. It is only when information is superimposed on a radio carrier wave that it truly becomes useful and fully functional. Likewise, it is only when information is superimposed on a stream of Chi that events, such as telepathic communication, clairvoyance, psychometry, etc., can take place.

The Aura

The aura is the subtle, yet readily viewable and palpable field of energetic energy generated by and surrounding, without exception, all matter, from the very simple to the very complex, both living and non-living. There are not only individual auras, but composite auras, as well. Entire mountains, for example, have auras composed of the collective energies of the rocks, soil, trees, snow, and everything that makes the mountain physically what it is.

Even our planet, the Earth, has an aura that is composed of the collective auras of everything that is found on and in it. Likewise, the aura of the human body is composite in nature, created not only by means of the energy produced through the various physiological energy-creating processes, such as digestion, respiration, et cetera, but also by the collective auras of its individual parts, from its simplest atoms and molecules through its varied and very complex organs.

Understand that every atom has an aura of its own and when atoms combine to form molecules, the aura of the molecule is composed of the combination of the auras of its atoms. It follows that the more complex a molecule is the greater is the energy of its aura, right?

Well, that depends on the energy levels of the atoms involved. The rule of thumb is: The more energy contained in the individual atoms, the more energy the molecule formed by those atoms will contain. During chemical reactions, there are exchanges of Chi that take place that vary the strength of the aura of the materials that are involved.

As you can see, the individual elements responsible for the creation of the auras surrounding all things can be quite complex and active.

Does the aura have a function?

Well, many people consider the aura to be an energy field surrounding a person that, through its various colors and densities, advertises that person's particular state of well-being, or that person's particular level of spiritual achievement. This, of course, is not a totally invalid understanding; it is, however, an incomplete one.

If we are trying to develop our psychic abilities properly, then a more complete understanding of the nature of our auras is required, or all efforts in the area of our psychic evolution will be, at best, very slow, and, in the end, may prove to be "ultimately" disappointing.

If we are to truly understand the nature of the aura, we must accept as axiomatic the fact that the aura is much more than just a barometer of the magnitude of a person's spiritual or emotional state. The fact is that the aura serves in human beings, as well as in all sentient life forms, as their very first line of defense.

"Understand that what the conscious mind is to the body, so the subconscious mind is to the aura."

That is, just as whatever comes into contact with our physical senses is automatically brought to the attention of our lower mind, whatever comes into contact with our aura is automatically brought to the attention of our higher mind. Just as any sort of intrusive physical contact with our body will cause our conscious mind to react in a defensive manner, any physical or energy contact made with our aura by an outside source will cause our subconscious mind to likewise act defensively.

This defensiveness, however, is not necessarily a universally good thing, for it becomes one of the most enormous impediments to the establishment of psychic liaisons between sentient beings. The reason why many mystics and those lay people who have tried to tap into their psychic powers have been disappointed with their efforts, is that they have not understood the protection that auras provide.

In a way, it is like attempting to break into your own home without first turning off the burglar alarm system and suddenly finding yourself face-to-face with a formidable team of security officers who prevent you from entering it. Knowing that this subconscious mind defense mechanism is in place, it is extremely important that you truly understand the nature of the aura in all of its aspects if you want to succeed in mastering your inner powers.

Chapter 2: Techniques to Mastering Energy

Normal Energy Expenditure

We, as living entities, are born with two energy reservoirs, one that determines the length of our lives, and the other that determines the quality of our days. The first reservoir is sealed and the energy spent cannot be replaced. As the energy level of this energetic reservoir declines over the course of our lives, our body ages and undergoes all of the natural changes associated with aging. When, at last, the energy level in this reservoir reaches the stage where it no longer contains enough to sustain the body, death occurs.

The second of our reservoirs is replenishable and our daily expenditures of energy require that we continuously replace as much of it as possible. This is accomplished through our natural bodily processes, such as the processing of food, respiration, sleep, association with other sentient beings, and even through our contact with inanimate objects. It is, in large part, the amount of energy contained in this reservoir that determines the amount of energy present in our auras at any particular time. When this reservoir is fully charged, our auras are at peak strength, and we experience a very real sense of health and well-being.

Conversely, when this reservoir is low, the strength and quality of our auras is weak. Varying levels of energy in this "restoreable" reservoir are normal in our daily lives and are generally nothing to be concerned about. However, when the energy level is critically low, there is a genuine cause for concern, for it may trigger a number of negative changes in our bodies, some of which may be tantamount to a physiological chain reaction, and may in their extreme be life threatening. This physiological chain reaction takes place because our higher minds respond to extemely low levels of energy by reprioritizing our body's energy expenditures.

That is, the energy distribution to the various organs of our bodies is shunted around and a new set of priorities is established. When energy levels are low, energy under the direction of the subconscious mind may be diverted away from certain non-essential organs and processes in order to maintain the minimum acceptable level of operation. Minimally, when this occurs we feel fatigued and are compelled to enter into a sleep or rest mode in order to replenish the energy necessary for acceptable bodily operation.

However, when the energy level of this reservoir is critically low, the restrictions the subconscious mind places on the organs of the body can be extreme and it will actually begin shutting down organs to the point where the situation may become life threatening. It may, for example, reduce the energy that it sends to the spleen, liver, pancreas, or kidneys. Or, it may even decrease the energy levels of the brain to the point where we are thrust into a state of coma. The subconscious mind does this in an effort to sustain life.

We have all experienced varying degrees of this shunting and reorganization of Chi at different times in our lives. Have you even been too tired to think? If you have, then you have experienced the higher mind shunting some Chi away from your brain in order to deliver that energy to another organ. When you reach such a state, it will clearly be reflected in the strength of your aura.

Simply stated, when your energetic level is high, your aura is strong and vibrant; when it is low, your aura becomes weak and appears irregular. The weaker your aura is, the more apt you are to suffer physically, and the less you will be able to defend yourself against psychic intrusion by outsiders.

The Presence of Danger

During times of danger, either real or imagined, the amount of Chi contained in our auras is automatically increased by the higher mind in order to strengthen our aura's defensive capabilities. This increase in energy not only increases the aura's overall sensitivity but also allows the aura to expand outwardly from the body without losing a great deal of density in the process.

This necessary expansion of the aura is controlled by the subconscious mind in order to increase its effective defensive range. The rule is: In times of safety, our aura's energy requirements are minimal and so the amount of energy that it contains is kept at normal levels; in times of danger (real or imagined), the aura enters a heightened defense mode and its energetic strength is augmented.

The Presence of Desease or Injury

When disease or injury is present in the body, Chi is sent by the subconscious mind to the afflicted area to help fight the disease and to make reparations to areas of damage. This process alters the distribution of energy in the aura.

For this reason, those well trained in certain esoteric fields of medicine can determine the presence of disease or injury in a patient by observing the various changes in quality [i.e., color, density, et cetera] present in their patient's aura. The rule is: When disease or injury is present in the body, the subconscious mind will increase the Chi to the affected area, and the strength of the aura surrounding the body will become imbalanced. That is, most of the aura may appear normal but there will be an increased density of Chi over the diseased or injured site. In extreme cases, the subconscious mind may even reduce the overall strength of the aura in order to use that Chi to fight a disease or repair an injury.

CONSCIOUS MIND THOUGHT

Our conscious mind is constantly affecting the strength and quality of our aura. The problem is that it does this in mostly negative ways. This means that our conscious mind is not necessarily always operating in our best interest. Our lower mind can, and often does, for example, waste enormous amounts of our Chi during the course of the day through its ceaseless and often useless chatter. It thinks about this and it thinks about that, worries about this and gets angry over that, and forms countless opinions about nearly everything that the physical senses come into contact with. This activity expends large quantities of our energy.

In many people, the unchecked activities of the conscious mind are one of the greatest causes of the energetic depletion of their auras. The reason for this is simple to understand: thinking requires energy. Of course, "not thinking" is not necessarily good either. The real problem is that the conscious mind engages in too much non-essential thought, and in particular, those non-essential thoughts that are emotion producing. Unchecked emotions sap the Chi in the energy reservoir and decrease the amount of Chi in the aura.

In addition, whenever our five physical senses come into contact with an external object, prompting the conscious mind to create a thought concerning that object, the subconscious mind immediately responds by creating a subconscious mind psychic conduit with the object. This results in a small but spontaneous transfer of Chi to the object.

Even if the subconscious mind psychic conduit lasts only a fraction of a moment, the loss of energy will still take place. Clearly, extraneous conscious mind thought is arguably the largest single non-physical factor affecting the magnitude and density of our auras. The remedy is meditation.

Meditation quiets the detrimental activities of the conscious mind. The proof lies in the fact that those who are engaged in daily regimens of meditation are very often seen to have denser and stronger auras than those who are not so engaged.

MIND STILLING TECHNIQUE

The Mind Stilling Technique is a way of taking immediate and decisive control of the conscious mind by stopping the myriad thoughts that interfere with not only our peace of mind, but our ability to tap into the rich areas of our psychic abilities.

[Step 1] Close your eyes and, exhaling through your nose, expel as much air from your lungs as you can. Hold your breath for a count of ten, or until your thoughts stop.

Note: *Observe what takes place when you hold your breath. Notice how the intensity and volume of your thoughts decrease, eventually disappearing entirely.*

[Step 2] Once your thoughts have stopped, begin a very slow, controlled, inhalation. Do not rush that first inhalation, even though you feel that you have to. Make every effort to control it. Fill your lungs to their normal capacity and hold your breath once again for a count of ten.

[Step 3] Then, exhale through your nose very slowly and empty your lungs of air, once again holding the extreme position for a count of ten before making another slow controlled inhalation. At this point, your conscious mind should be calm and uncluttered. You may repeat this exercise as many times as necessary.

YIN CHI INFUSION TECHNIQUE

The Yin chi infusion technique, is one of the most extraordinary techniques that we found for the quieting of the conscious mind. It may be performed in a meditation posture, sitting in a chair, lying on a bed, or even while standing. If performed correctly, it will quiet the lower mind in less than a minute.

[Step 1] Do a complete exhalation through your nose, exhaling as much air out of your lungs as you can and then hold your breath for a count of five.

[Step 2] Now, you must fill your entire body with Chi. To do this, first imagine that your entire body is hollow... arms, legs, torso, everything. Perform a complete inhalation, following your Chi-laden breath with your mind's eye as it enters you, filling your body completely, from the tip of your toes to the top of your head.

[Step 3] Place the palm of your right hand over your Heart Vortex, located over your heart [the area in the center of your chest] and exhale through your nose, following breath as it travels up from your "hollow" feet, through the center of your "hollow" body, down through your "hollow" right arm, out of your palm, and into your Heart Vortex. Repeat this technique one to three times, as needed. It may, of course, be repeated as many times as necessary.

Variation: *Another variation is to entwine your hands as if praying and place them on the chest and proceed as mentioned above. To change the energy and feeling, you may also cross the feet with left on top and then right foot on top. By just changing the feet you get a different experience.*

Seeing The Aura

[Step 1] Take a small potted plant and place it on a table in front of a light-colored background, preferably white.

[Step 2] Position yourself approximately three to four feet away from the plant and quiet you conscious mind utilizing the Yin chi infusion technique.

[Step 3] Once you have quieted your conscious mind, stare into the center of the plant's foliage. In only moments, you will see a subtle glow surrounding the leaves and stem of the plant. That is the plant's aura.

Exercise 2

[Step 1] After successfully completing exercise 1, pull a leaf from the plant and place it and the plant on the table on a black or white piece of paper or a black or white tablecloth.

[Step 2] Use the Yin chi infusion technique to quiet your lower mind.

[Step 3] Observe the leaf carefully and you will see the aura surrounding it. However, there is more to see. If you look very carefully, you will also see a narrow column of indigo-colored Chi extending from the leaf to the plant.

Exercise 3

[Step 1] Have a friend stand in front of a white wall. Position yourself approximately four to five feet away.

[Step 2] Quiet your conscious mind by utilizing the Yin chi infusion technique.

[Step 3] Once your mind is quiet, look at her or him, paying particular attention to the edges of their body. You should be able to see your friend's aura.

Auric Massage- For Couples

[Step 1] In a candle lit room, have your partner lie on their back on a bed and relax. They may have their eyes open or closed; it's purely optional. For the best results, your partner should be clad in as little clothing as possible. Here, of course, you should let your level of comfort be your guide.

[Step 2] Both you and your partner should quiet your conscious minds utilizing the Yin chi infusion technique.

[Step 3] Kneel beside your partner and place the aura surrounding the relaxed palms of your hands on the surface of the aura on either side of their face. As soon as you do, they should feel heat and a slight tingling on their face.

[Step 4] Very slowly, begin to move your hands over your partner's entire aura, lingering as long as you like over the more sensual areas of the body. Wherever your aura touches your partner's aura, heat and tingling will be experienced. The rest I will leave to your imagination. I am sure that you will know what to do from there.

Auric Lie Detector- *When lying the aura will expand and become brighter and denser*

[Step 1] Have a friend stand in front of a light-colored wall.

[Step 2] Stand approximately five feet away and quiet your conscious mind utilizing the Yin chi infusion technique.

[Step 3] Looking along the edges of their body, view their aura, paying particular attention to its depth and density.

[Step 4] Ask your friend a few questions that you already know the answers to. If they answer truthfully, you will see no changes in their aura.

[Step 5] When you are ready, tell your friend to give a false answer to any question that they choose to lie about. Then, ask your questions. When they lie, you will immediately see a marked change in the depth and density of their aura.

Exercise #2 for Lie Detector

[Step 1] Have a friend stand in front of a light-colored wall.

[Step 2] Stand approximately five feet away and quiet your conscious mind utilizing the Yin chi infusion technique.

[Step 3] View their aura, paying particular attention to its depth and density.

[Step 4] Now, ask your friend questions that you do not have the answers to and see what happens. It is important for you to understand that when a person is asked a question that causes them discomfort, their aura may appear to pulsate slightly. This pulsation should not be interpreted as lying. Lying is indicated solely by a marked increase in both auric density and depth.

Chapter 3: Telepathy, Transmitting Thoughts

Telepathy

Simply, telepathy is the transmission of thought, however subtle that thought may be, from one living being to another. It is the most common and natural of our inner powers and takes place all around us, all the time, in every conceivable combination. That is, man transmits to animals, animals-to-man, man-to-plants, plants-to-man, animals-to-plants, plants-to-animals, man-to-man, animal-to-animal, plant-to-plant, and so on.

If this is true and telepathic communications are so widespread, then we could ask: why does telepathic reception seem so completely beyond the capacity of most of us to experience in our daily lives?

This is certainly a fair question, one that crosses a skeptic's mind every time the subject is broached. The answer is that there are two factors chiefly responsible for our inability to experience the plethora of telepathic communications taking place around us: our lower minds and our auras.

First, as to our conscious minds, it is evident that the enormous evolutionary strides that we have undergone as human beings have brought us into a state where our conscious minds have become so developed, so dominant, that they have become the principal mental voice in our lives. We experience this dominance constantly throughout the course of our day.

But there was a time in man's distant past, before the conscious mind took this dominant position, that our subconscious mind ruled and telepathy played an enormous role in our ability to not only communicate with others, but aided us enormously in understanding and living in harmony with the living elements of our environment. This gave us a sense of naturalness and oneness with all of nature, something that seems to be sadly missing among the majority of people today.

In a very real sense our evolved, noisy, discriminating, conscious minds took our once natural and much used telepathic abilities and simply covered them over. It did this so well and so subtly over time, that today it is not uncommon for many people casually hearing the phrase "telepathic communication" to immediately reduce it to nothing more than an amusing and idle speculation.

Since our telepathic apparatus lies deep within the recesses of our subconscious mind, it is not difficult to understand why the presently dominant conscious mind has little understanding of it and why it would doubt its existence. It is rather ironic to think that the conscious mind, that very component of us responsible in large part for the disappearance of such a useful and natural ability as telepathy, should today find the very idea of its existence so odd and alien.

The second part of the answer has to do with the protective presence of our auras, a mechanism that is as simple as it is, by nature, ingenious. It not only protects us from the constantly radiated intrusive thoughts of others but also effectively interferes with the ability of others to receive our thoughts.

Imagine the enormous difficulty a radio receiver would have receiving signals if a powerful electrical field surrounded it. That electrical field would effectively block reception, wouldn't it? This is precisely what our auras do. That is, they effectively block telepathic transmissions from reaching us. Our experience has taught us that when our lower minds are quiet enough and the strength of our auras is reduced to relatively low levels, then telepathic communication is not only possible, but becomes relatively easy to perform.

This is why you must increase the overall sensitivity of your chi to be able to tune into all of the vibrations that can be received by you at any given time.

How We Think

To understand telepathy, we must understand how we think. Well, to begin with, as sophisticated as our conscious mind prides itself to be, for the most part we think mainly in pictures.

That is, our conscious mind takes sensory information presented to it by the body's various physical sense faculties and then quickly, almost instantaneously, creates a picture based on that data. It then searches its memory for previously recorded information associated with that image. If, for example, we see or hear the word elephant, what comes to our mind?

Yes, we see the image of an elephant. If we see or hear the word zebra, likewise we see the image of a zebra, stripes, and all. In both of these cases, the most immediate information available to us would be the picture of an elephant or zebra that has been previously recorded on our conscious mind memories.

It is generally only after that happens that other more specific information comes, such as any particular statistical information that we may possess concerning elephants or zebras, such as the animal's height, weight, disposition, and any past personal contacts we may have had with the animal. Of course, if we had never seen or heard of an elephant or zebra before, no such picture would appear on the screen of our conscious minds and the word elephant or zebra would be seem meaningless.

Even so, knowing that they were animals is enough to trigger our conscious mind into searching its memory banks and presenting us with a collage of pictures of animals that may be to some extent analogous. In such a case, instead of summoning an image of a zebra, for instance, it may project to us the image of a horse. No, it is not a zebra, but it is pretty close. This is an example of associative thinking and is important in understanding the telepathic process.

Another example of how the mind thinks in pictures has to do with the conscious retrieval of memories. If we were asked to think back to a particular event or time in our life, for example, what would run through our lower mind? That's right, pictures, images of our childhood, or when we graduated high school, or when we were married. Whatever words we do come up with are generally not actually part of the memory at all, but are merely superimposed interpretations of those pictures, biased comments created by our conscious mind.

Understand that it is not that the conscious mind cannot or does not think in the abstract, certainly it does. It reasons, describes, and generally gives consideration to ideas based on whatever external sensory information it receives before it vocalizes those thoughts internally to us.

This, of course, is a much more sophisticated process than merely thinking in pictures and is really the only ability that our human conscious mind has that distinguishes it from the purely picture-thinking processes that occur in most of the lower animal kingdom. Even so, our conscious mind still

76

favors thinking in pictures, which is fortunate because it is the easiest form of thought to transmit telepathically.

TELEPATHY & THE AURA

Every sentient being [i.e. plants, animals, and humanity] is constantly transmitting its picture-thoughts to the rest of the world in waves much like those generated by a radio transmitter. If this is so, then it could be asked: why is it that, if we are surrounded by so much telepathic activity, that we aren't constantly bombarded by a cacophony of chaotic and maddening picture-thoughts, a huge number of which would have associative emotions attached to them?

The answer is that we are, in fact, constantly bombarded by myriad telepathic thoughts; however, the reason why many of us are unaware of them is to be found in our own human evolution.

The rule is: The higher in the evolutionary ladder we ascend, the more insulation is present to block out the countless extraneous and, often, intrusive telepathic thoughts that relentlessly assail us.

Yes, we might think that the constant chatter going on inside our conscious mind is the sort of protection from telepathic intrusion that we are referring to, but it would be wrong to think that. Our conscious mind chatter is certainly interference, but definitely not protection. The fact is that the conscious mind cannot, regardless of how much chattering it does, prevent us from receiving telepathic messages; it simply interferes with our awareness of them.

Our real protection from intrusive telepathic thought is provided by a mechanism that is as simple as it is, by nature, ingenious. It is our aura. It not only protects us from the constantly radiated intrusive thoughts of others but also effectively prevents others from receiving our thoughts.

Again, imagine the enormous difficulty a radio receiver would have receiving signals if a large electrical field surrounded it. That electrical field would effectively block reception. That is precisely what our auras do. Therefore, if we want to engage in meaningful telepathic communication with others, the careful control of both our own aura and theirs is a necessity. In later lessons, you will learn how to do this.

MORE TELEPATHY BASICS

In order for useful telepathic transmission to take place, there are two fundamental conditions that have to be met. The first is that the amount of Chi present in the sender's aura must be raised to peak levels. The second is that the person who is to receive the telepathic message has either a reduced amount of Chi in their aura and/or willingly allows an open-gated subconscious mind psychic conduit to be established between him and the sender.

Regarding the first condition, just as in radio broadcasting, the stronger the radio signal is the stronger and clearer the reception will be. Similarly, the more empowered our auras are with Chi, the more powerful become our personal telepathic transmitters. In times of crises, for example, we become virtual powerhouses of telepathic thought transmission because during those times the amount of Chi in our aura is automatically increased by our subconscious mind much beyond its normal levels.

Because of this enhancement, when we are in distress, we become like powerful radio transmitters broadcasting our distress calls to the rest of the world. This is a normal response to crises and not at all something that should be considered odd or abnormal. This is the reason why we hear of so many documented stories of people in peril making their predicament telepathically known to others, especially to those with whom they share an open subconscious mind psychic conduit at the time, such as those that exist between a person and their close friends and relatives.

This is how it works: The increase of Chi in the aura, the establishment of psychic conduits or paths, and the opening and closing of psychic gates, are all orchestrated by the subconscious mind. In times of great peril, the subconscious mind diverts Chi away from various internal bodily functions and delivers it to the aura in order to enhance the aura's protective and telepathic broadcasting capabilities.

It then sends out a distress call comprised primarily of information relevant to the nature and pertinent conditions of the situation. The problem is, however, that because of the natural protective barriers created by their own auras, vast majorities of the seeming limitless number of possible receivers simply do receive it, while those who do receive it either have open-gated subconscious mind psychic conduits established with the sender or are in a physical or mental state where the strength of their aura is, at that moment, greatly reduced.

INVOLUNTARY TELEPATHIC COMMUNICATION

Involuntary telepathic communications are those instances of telepathic sending or receiving, which occurs naturally and spontaneously in our life. It is really the rule and not the exception. That is, again, we must understand that there are natural telepathic communications occurring constantly between all sentient entities-between people, animals, and plants-in all the possible combinations.

However, during times of great stress, especially during those times where safety is a major factor, the subconscious mind by design automatically increases the amount of Chi in our aura to what can be considered broadcast levels, turning a person, animal, or even a plant, into a redoubtable and powerful telepathic transmitter, broadcasting a wide-ranging distress calls to any and all parties who may possibly be summoned for aid.

Certainly, we are all familiar with at least a few of the many stories of people who have been saved from danger and even death by psychically communicating the particulars of their predicaments to others. Just as there are times when we are excellent involuntary telepathic senders, there are natural, yet odd, moments in our life when we become superb involuntary psychic receivers. There are four reasons responsible for this:

[1] Because our conscious mind happens to be unusually tranquil and we feel a very real sense of serenity and safety. When this happens, our subconscious mind responds by decreasing the amount of Chi in our aura. This effectively lowers our defenses and makes us more receptive to telepathic messages.

[2] Because our conscious mind is so quiet, there is simply less noisy interference offered to telepathic reception at the conscious mind level.

[3] Our conscious mind, being serene, is doing nothing to trigger our subconscious mind into taking defensive action.

[4] We may already have natural open-gated subconscious mind psychic conduits established with the sender.

A typical example of involuntary telepathic communication is between family members or those we love. Understand that because an open-gated subconscious mind psychic conduit normally exists between parents and their children, a son or daughter's cry for her/his mother can be automatically transmitted through that conduit. It just happens involuntarily and naturally.

How often has this happened to you?

How often has just thinking about a person prompted them to call you? This is another example of involuntary telepathy. Certainly, unless you were well versed in the process, the idea of contacting that person telepathically had never entered your mind and yet there it was . . .

Telepathic communication. As often occurs with many people, our first instinct is to label it as nothing more than a coincidence. This is a natural reaction, but is it really just a coincidence? No, clearly, it is not a coincidence at all, especially if we consider the odds of something like that happening. Again, we must understand that because of the already established higher mind psychic conduit existing, the thought of a phone call is passed from one person to the other.

Since the idea of a phone call coming in from someone we know, or one that we make ourselve, thinking, that the thought is our own, and so we act upon it. It makes us wonder how many thoughts that we have acted on in the past were not even our own thoughts, doesn't it?

We often make the mistake of believing that our private thoughts are just that, our private thoughts, and that they are immune from violation or intrusion from the outside. This, naturally, is what most people believe, however, it could not be further from the truth. The reality is that we are transmitting our private thoughts all the time and that we are often subjected to any of the consequences that those private thoughts might provoke when picked up by others.

Even if the letter of those thoughts are only picked up by another person's subconscious mind and not relayed word-for-word to their lower minds, the sense of those thoughts will cause them to respond in one way or another, either negatively or positively.

This is, in part, the nature of the world we inhabit and the nature of the extrasensory telepathic powers that we all possess. Therefore, to ignore these powers or to disregard even the possibility that they exist is definitely not in our best interest. So, like Jerry, how many times have you destroyed sales? In fact, how many times have you destroyed friendships and relationships without being aware of it? Remember, private thoughts are not really quite as private as you believe they are.

On the whole, involuntary telepathic communication is just that, spontaneous and unplanned; a communication that normally occurs in the blink of an eye and often has both of the participants wondering who had had the original thought. For example, how often have you and a person that you were with said the exact same thing at the exact same time?

Think about it for a moment and I am sure that you will be able to recall a number of those incidents, especially, with someone that you were near to, such as a spouse, sibling, a close friend, or one of your children. When it happened, did you think it was a coincidence?

Well, the odds of two people saying the exact same thing at the exact same time, you have to admit, is pretty remote and well beyond chance.

Another very common example of involuntary telepathic communication is, believe it or not, yawning. Certainly, you've heard the expression: yawning is contagious. How many times in your life did you find yourself yawning at the same time the person you were with yawned or vice versa? Was it just a coincidence? No, not really, it was the product of involuntary telepathic communication.

Understand that when you are tired, your conscious mind quiets down and that brings your subconscious mind forward. Since it is the subconscious mind that is responsible for the maintenance of the body, should it require a brief increase in oxygen, it will produce a yawn. Since subconscious minds between friends and relatives normally and quite naturally establish open-gated psychic conduits with each other, the idea of a yawn is something that is easily transferred telepathically. The next time this happens to you, barring coincidence, you should realize that you just had a genuine telepathic experience.

INVOLUNTARY TELEPATHIC COMMUNICATION & THE EMOTIONS

Thoughts are not the only things transferred telepathically between sentient beings; the emotions are also communicated in this way. Telepathically transmitted feelings of love, hate, revulsion, fear, attraction, envy, pity, distrust, and others, are often the cause of not only the establishment and sustaining of relationships and other interactions taking place between people, but, unfortunately, are also responsible for the many of the negative qualities inherent in relationships, as well. Therefore, it is not just what we say or think that is communicated to the other party during a conversation, but what we feel is also transferred.

Sensing The Loving Feelings of Another

Something that is quite common in many relationships, is even if all of the necessary outward elements seem to be in place, there is still communication taking place on a subconscious mind level that can tell us that there is "Something is missing." Of course, there are times when the opposite is true.

That is, when, although there are outward signs that are telling us that something is missing, what is being involuntarily transmitted telepathically to us are emotional elements telling us that perhaps the other person does, in fact, really and truly love us. Bearing this in mind, it does not pay for us to allow ourselves to make judgments based only on what we see or hear coming from the other person, but those judgments should take into consideration what is going on behind the scenes, what they are thinking and feeling, as well.

Projecting a Negative Energy

Some people want one thing but project another. Many want relationship, job, business, health success on the outside, but the energy they project is totally different. How was it clear to us? Because of negative situations in our past, sometimes our mind begins to project those feelings as a defense mechanism against the possibility of a similar situation from ever happening again. Apparently, the negative images that are broadcast is the mind's way of protecting us.

The telepathic defense mechanism is in place and functions to assist us from danger. Often times it interprets feelings from the past and installs it into the present to keep us from harm, rejection or danger.

How to Clear The Mind of Self- Sabotaging Energy

1. You must face and come to terms with the issues of the past and let them go.
2. You must replace the negative image in your mind with the positive image you desire to be true.

THE RULES CONCERNING SUBCONSCIOUS MIND PSYCHIC CONDUITS

The first rule tells us that mutually deep-seated feelings of attachment or rapport typified by emotions such as love, offer us a perfectly natural, positive climate for the establishment of open-gated subconscious mind psychic conduits and the free exchange of subconscious mind-to-subconscious mind information.

We see examples of this all of the time, as in the case of a married couple, or any group of people for that matter, who have been together for a number of years and have a relationship that has become a comfortable one, especially where feelings of love and trust exist.

Under these conditions, the gates on both sides of all established subconscious mind psychic conduits are generally open and the subconscious mind psychic conduits are operational. This explains why, over time, the parties involved in these relationships become so mutually intuitive toward each other. A married couple, for example, with open-gated subconscious mind psychic conduits operating between them seem to be quite well informed as to what is taking place mentally and emotionally inside of each other.

Here we find that it is often displayed whenever both parties say or do the exact same thing at the very same time. The second rule can be considered the prime reason why telepathic communication has declined to virtual latency in the present state of human evolution and why it has reached the point where any exhibited telepathic talents are treated as peculiar deviations from the norm, rather than a common and readily accepted part of human life.

There is much distrust and enmity existing between people in the world today. When we consider that we have the automatic and natural ability to open or close the gates on our side of a subconscious mind psychic conduit, protecting us not only from unwanted social relationships, but from unwanted psychic intrusions, it is no wonder why telepathic communication among humans seem to have declined in modern times.

When we consider our own personal conscious mind thoughts, associative feelings, and personal reactions to the people we know, the people we love, hate or fear, and the strangers we meet, then we can gain an instant insight into how we personally manage our own psychic gates.

Whenever we experience a sense of distance between ourselves and another person, for example, we can be certain that one or possibly both of our subconscious mind psychic gates are closed. Conversely, when we experience warmth and closeness between ourselves and another person, we can be sure that both gates are open, allowing not only the free exchange of Chi or energy between us, but also the unencumbered exchange of telepathic information. This, of course, is what we would need to happen if we wanted to establish telepathic or clairvoyant communication with another person.

TELEPATHIC THOUGHT RECEIVING

As to condition one, understand that both the higher and conscious mind have an enormous influence on the strength of our aura and must be brought under our control so that our aura offers as little resistance as possible to telepathic thought reception.

The rule is: *the more defensive our lower mind is towards a sender, the more Chi our subconscious mind will inject into our aura in order to protect us against them.*

Therefore, if we have conscious mind thoughts or feelings that contain elements of fear, suspicion, anxiety, hatred, et cetera, concerning the sender then we can be sure that our higher mind has already responded and increased the amount of Chi in our aura as a protective measure.

It does this in order to make our aura more sensitive and impenetrable to psychic intrusion effectively taking away from us the first requirement for good telepathic reception. This defensive action, in turn, automatically prompts the subconscious mind to close its gate at its end of whatever subconscious mind psychic conduit the sender has established [or is trying to establish] with us.

This, of course, effectively destroys the second condition. As we see, the first two conditions are closely related. It is like a mini-chain reaction. In order to reverse the process and reduce the strength of our aura while simultaneously making sure that the gate at our end of the subconscious mind psychic conduit remains open, we have to eliminate our fears, suspicions, hatreds, et cetera concerning the sender.

There are two relatively easy methods to do this.

The first, although not necessarily the best, is to reason-out a trust with the sender. That is, to intentionally and wholeheartedly place our trust in the person that we are allowing into to our sanctum sanctorum, our inner world. We can choose, of course, to simply work with a person that we have known for a long time, one with whom we already have a friendly, trusting, relationship.

This is the best way, especially for beginners. The drawback, however, is that it greatly limits the number of senders that we can voluntarily receive from.

The second method and one that is, for many reasons, superior to the first, is to enter into a state where our conscious mind is serenely at ease. That is, to enter a state of superlative quietude where the conscious mind is so calm, so untroubled, that it is unable or unwilling to prompt the subconscious mind into defensively increasing the Chi of our aura or closing our psychic gate.

Mastering the **Mind Stilling technique**, **Yin chi infusion technique**, and other meditative techniques can bring this about. Once our conscious mind is quiet enough, there is less of a tendency for it to superimpose information on the telepathic messages we receive.

This nicely satisfies the third condition. Clearly, all three conditions for good telepathic reception are linked. The quieter our conscious mind is, the less we are apt to reject the sender by increasing the strength of our aura, closing our psychic gate, or superimposing our own thoughts on those we are receiving. Therefore, the key to good telepathic thought reception is good meditative technique

GENERAL THOUGHT RECEPTION EXERCISE

[Step 1] Place yourself in a room that is free from noise and other distractions, a room that has an atmosphere that promotes as little physical sensory stimulation as possible.

[Step 2] Assume a comfortable position. You may sit on a chair, or even lay down on a bed or the floor, if you like.

[Step 3] Perform the Mind Stilling technique followed by the Yin chi infusion technique.

[Step 4] Once your conscious mind is quiet, have a sense of sanctioning the reception of any and all incoming psychic transmissions, regardless of their content.

[Step 5] With your eyes closed, allow your mind to pass through the "3rd Eye" [located in the center of your forehead between and slightly above your eyebrows] and deep into the void beyond. Continue traveling deeper and deeper until you encounter an image. You are now receiving telepathically. Remember, people generally think in picture-words and that those images represent thoughts and ideas.

[Step 6] When you are ready to stop receiving, simply bring yourself out of it by stimulating your conscious mind with sensory input, such as rubbing your face, turning on a light, playing some music, or washing your face.

TARGETED THOUGHT RECEPTION

Picture the person in your minds eye and grasp a concept of communication with them.

TECHNIQUE

[Step 1] Place yourself in a room that is free from noise and other distractions.

[Step 2] You may assume sit comfortably in a meditation posture, sit on a chair or sofa, or lie down on a bed.

[Step 3] Use the Mind Stilling technique followed by the Yin chi infusion technique, to quiet your conscious mind.

[Step 4] Picture the person that you want to receive the telepathic transmissions from. You must see them clearly in your mind's eye. To help you do this, a photograph of the person would be useful. Picturing the person will generate a narrow stream of Chi to the aura of that person and establish the necessary psychic conduit with them. You will know that open-gated contact has been established between you when you feel a subtle release of pressure in the area of your aura just in front of your "3rd Eye", located in the center of your forehead between your eyebrows.

[Step 5] Once you feel that the subconscious mind psychic conduit has been establish with the subject, enter through your "3rd Eye", and travel deep into the void beyond. Continue traveling until you encounter an image. If possible, try to understand that image before going deeper and encountering other images.

[Step 6] When you are ready to stop receiving, simply bring yourself out of it by stimulating your conscious mind with sensory input, such as rubbing your face, turning on a light, playing some music, et cetera.

TRANSMISSION OF TELEPATHIC THOUGHT

In order for us to transmit telepathic thought effectively, the amount of Chi in our aura must be raised to what can be called broadcast levels.

The rule is: *The more empowered our aura is, the easier it is for us to transmit telepathic thought.*

There are two ways in which this can be achieved, Spontaneous and Induced. An understanding of both methods is paramount to achieving the sort of power necessary to command this very useful telepathic ability. Understand that the emotions created in us by our conscious mind are among the primary factors determining the strength of our aura during the course of our day.

This means that our emotions and our natural ability to transmit telepathically are linked. In fact, it would be fair to say that the state of our emotions is the single most influential factor in the creation of spontaneous or natural telepathic transmitting. If we are in a state of immanent fear, for example, a condition where we are in great fear for our life, our subconscious mind will automatically direct enough Chi to our aura to reinforce not only its defensive capabilities but to increase its ability to transmit telepathic distress calls.

Of course, it is not recommended that we intentionally place ourselves in a life-threatening situation just so that we can practice communicating telepathically with the rest of the sentient world.

Would it work?

Yes, certainly, it would work, but what would be the point of risking our lives just so we could practice telepathically screaming for help? It just would not make sense, especially when we can safely raise the magnitude of Chi in our aura to broadcast levels simply by employing techniques designed to increase the Chi.

Increasing the Chi in our aura by employing them will enable us to transmit induced or controlled telepathic thought without all of the fuss and danger associated with the often-bizarre emotional methods of aura strengthening practiced elsewhere. Again, during a life or death situation, telepathic transmissions will occur naturally and automatically and not much, if anything, has to be done in order to transmit effectively.

Why?

Because life and death situations have a tendency to panic the conscious mind, causing the subconscious mind respond to that panic by increasing the strength of the aura in order to assure that there is enough Chi to psychically transmit the necessary distress calls. This sort of subconscious mind response to immanent danger is not limited just to us, but is universal throughout both the animal and plant kingdoms.

EXERCISE #1 MEETING HALF WAY

[Step 1] Have your partner sit across from you and quiet their conscious mind using the Mind Stilling technique followed by the Yin chi infusion technique in order to help make them more receptive.

[Step 2] Build your Aura circulating your chi in a clockwise rotational pattern. It may be helpful to do several minutes of "Blood Washing" to get the desired effect.

[Step 3] Have a picture of an object that you want to transmit in front of you. Stare at it until, when you close your eyes you can see the image clearly in your mind's eye. When you are ready, enter deep into your "3rd Eye" and picture the image there.

Note: *In the beginning, it may be easier to start with a simple shape, such as a square, star, triangle, et cetera, rather than a more complicated image, such as landscape or intricate pattern. Naturally, as you become more successful with the technique, you can gradually introduce more complex and diverse images.*

[Step 4] Have your partner enter the subconscious mind psychic conduit established between you through their "3rd Eye" and travel until they reach the image suspended in the void.

EXERCISE #2 SENDING IT ALL THE WAY

[Step 1] Have your partner sit across from you and quiet their conscious mind using the Mind Stilling technique followed by the Yin chi infusion technique to make them more receptive.

[Step 2] Build Your Chi like in the exercise before

[Step 3] Have a picture of the object that you want to transmit in front of you; a simple shape would do for a beginning. Stare at the image until, when you close your eyes, you can see it clearly in your mind's eye. When you are ready, enter in through your "3rd Eye" and picture the image there. Once it is firmly established, have the sense of propelling that image deep into the void of the psychic conduit until you feel a very subtle release of pressure. This release of pressure indicates that you have passed through their psychic gate. They should now be in receipt of that image.

[Step 4] Have your partner close their eyes and, practicing their reception technique, tell you what they see.

AURA TO AURA CONTACT

[Step 1] Have your partner sit across the table from you with their eyes closed and have them quiet their conscious mind using the Mind Stilling technique followed by the Yin chi infusion technique.

[Step 2] Build Your Chi utilizing the Blood Washing Method

[Step 3] Lightly hold your partner's hands in your own.

[Step 4] Stare at the picture until, when you close your eyes you can see the image clearly in your mind's eye. When you are ready, enter in through your "3rd Eye", and place the image there, sending it deep into the void.

[Step 5] Now, have your partner enter the subconscious mind psychic conduit through their "3rd Eye" and retrieve the image.

SENDING THOUGHTS TO AN UNSUSPECTING PERSON

[Step 1] Think of the person that you want to transmit to. This will automatically establish the subconscious mind psychic conduit between you. A photograph of the person would be helpful.

[Step 2] A good rapport between you and the receiver must then be established. To do this you must make every effort to assure that your initial telepathic contact is as benign and non-aggressive as possible

[Step 3] You must have a clear image of just what it is that you want to transmit. Make sure that you do not confuse the receiver with picture-words that appear in your mind that have nothing to do with the message that you want them to receive. It could, for example, be the image of them placing a phone call to you.

[Step 4] Once you have the image clearly in your mind's eye, enter the void through your "3rd Eye" and place the image there. Then, project it deep into the void until you feel a subtle release of pressure.

APPEARING AT 2 PLACES AT THE SAME TIME

[Step 1] Build your chi

[Step 2] Visualize exactly whom you wish to use as the subject or distant receiver of this technique. Initially, you should choose someone with whom you already have an established open-gated subconscious mind psychic conduit, such as a close friend or relative, otherwise, you may have to employ a gate-opening technique, which for the beginner would simply be complicating a reasonable straightforward task. Naturally, once you have this technique perfected, you may elect to expand it to include those with whom you do not share a pre-existing open-gated psychic conduit.

[Step 3] Project the picture or image of you standing in front of the receiver through your "3rd Eye" and deep into the void of the subconscious mind psychic conduit between you.

Note: *It is better for beginners to keep their technique as simple as possible. That is, just appearing in front of the subject should be enough to create the desired effect. This may be expanded later to include whatever physical movements and actions you may choose to present to the subject or subjects.*

[Step 4] Merely sending the receiver the image of you standing in front of them is not enough. There must be correlative auric pressure to accompany the thought. This tactile sensation will take it out of the realm of just mental imagery and lend it a reality that the receiver's subconscious mind will identify with and accept. To do this, the imaging that you are sending must include you standing before them looking at a particular part of the receiver's body. I suggest staring at his or her face because it will seem most natural.

Note: *By sending the image of you standing before the receiver staring at their face, you will actually be creating a second subconscious mind psychic conduit that will transfer Chi that contacts the receiver's aura there. This auric contact will create a convincing pressure on the receiver's aura, completing the illusion. In other words, to be convincing, both what the receiver sees and what he or she feels must tell them that you are really there.*

[1] Any negative thought on your part will automatically cause the subject to close their end of the psychic conduit and prevent the technique from being successful. Therefore, all negative thoughts you have that may cause them to do that must be avoided.

[2] The amount of Chi that you transfer when you make contact with the receiver's aura must be kept to a minimum. That is, it should just be enough to stimulate their aura and no more. It must also be Yin Chi, that feels euphoric and blissful. Too much Chi striking the subject's aura will cause their subconscious mind to treat it as a threat, which will cause them to defend against the intrusion by closing the gate on their side of the subconscious mind psychic conduit.

[3] It is advisable to conduct this technique in a quiet room, one that, aside from the witnesses present, is free from noise and other distractions. Do not become discouraged if, at first, you have difficulty with this technique. Never be in a rush toward mastery; it takes time, patience, and practice.

Chapter 4: Clairvoyance, Seeing The Unseen

CLAIRVOYANCE

The existence of subconscious mind psychic conduits give rise, in many people, to the notion of a universal mind at work in varying degrees between all beings. This is understandable. In truth, however, at the subconscious mind level, the universal mind exists, as a direct connection to God. We do not find what is tantamount to a universal mind until we reach the soul level, where devoid of all impediments and subjective biases, we arrive at our true essence and experience the oneness of all things through God The Father.

Understand that at the subconscious mind level of consciousness instead of one commonly shared perception of existence, we have many, as many as there are living beings, each with individual experiences, histories, and personal biases. What gives rise to the notion that the subconscious mind is synonymous with a universal mind comes from the propensity that the subconscious mind has for creating psychic links or conduits with other subconscious minds.

This gives us an indefatigable sense of personal expansion, one that seems limitless but really isn't. What gives us this sense of universality is the fact that a single person can have an enormous number of subconscious mind conduits in place with other sentient beings who, in turn, also have in place a vast number of psychic subconscious mind conduits with many other sentient beings.

As a result, we find ourselves psychically linked to others both directly and indirectly. Consequently, it is no small wonder that those of us who travel through this seemingly endless web of psychic connections see this as the ultimate experience of universal mind with God.

In order to travel through all of the subconscious mind psychic conduits of the maze, all of the gates on both ends of all of those conduits have to be open and therefore operational. If one or more of the psychic gates are closed, then our psychic journey in that particular direction is ended and we must either find a new route or somehow find a way to open those closed gates.

Because of this, we find that our voyages through these subconscious mind networks and our ability to gather information fall short of that which we would expect from a true communication with God, which again, is normally only found at the soul level. Even so, although the subconscious mind and its associated climes are not the ultimate level of awareness possible for us, it is certainly massive steps up from the sparse opportunities presented to us by our limited and error-prone conscious minds.

INVOLUNTARY SUBCONSCIOUS MIND CLAIRVOYANCE

Of the two types of involuntary subconscious mind clairvoyance, receptive and projected, receptive is the least common, even though the seemingly numerous stories we hear from time to time involving this type of clairvoyance might have us believing otherwise.

Involuntary subconscious mind clairvoyant experiences are produced in times of great stress; times when immanent danger prompts the subconscious mind of a person to reach out for assistance; to transmit a frantic, panic-ridden, distress-laden telepathic message, hoping against hope for an immediate, peril dispelling response.

In fact, it is not unlike a S.O.S. distress call sent out by a ship at sea when it finds itself imperiled; a call that is directed to any and all vessels in the vicinity that might be able to render aid. This being the case, it is not at all uncommon for individuals totally unfamiliar to the subject to receive this psychic cry for help, especially since the maze of subconscious mind psychic conduits available to it at the time may be quite extensive.

Yet, those that are emotionally closest to the distressed subject are generally the ones most likely to experience it. This is so because the relationship already has open-gated subconscious mind psychic conduits directly and firmly in place and functioning, allowing for an unimpeded exchange of telepathic information.

In receptive involuntary subconscious mind clairvoyance, as with all forms of clairvoyance, the receiver essentially shares all of the sender's visual, auditory, emotional, and tactile experiences occurring at the time. There are many examples of this, such as that of a mother who unexpectedly is thrust into the perilous circumstances her child is undergoing at the moment.

Here, suddenly, without warning, she is seeing, hearing, and feeling all of the physical and emotional elements of her child's difficulty. This form of clairvoyance may rightfully be regarded as a form of involuntarily induced astral projection, a sort of astral kidnapping, since she is abruptly transported against her will from her reality to that of her child's.

What allows this to happen is the naturally open-gated subconscious mind psychic conduit existing between them. Interestingly, with the vast open-gated subconscious mind psychic conduit networking in place at any one time throughout the world, there are instances that occur where the closest person is subtly bypassed and one or more people somewhere down the sender's psychic conduit complex are contacted.

This occurrence is not as rare as we might think. Of course, it could also happen that the closest person is in fact contacted, as well as one or more other people in the psychic maze.

When this happens, because the recipient's subconscious mind psychic conduit network is always different than that of the sender, one or more of the recipients of the clairvoyant experience may be totally unknown to the sender.

Therefore, as we see, through subconscious mind psychic linking, there is the potential for an enormous range of possibilities, a massive number of possible psychic contacts. It should be noted that involuntary receptive higher mind clairvoyant experiences are totally devoid of any prophetic content and deal only with the matter at hand.

That is, they are not addressing future or past events, but are limited to incidents that are taking place at the present time. <u>There is a second form of receptive involuntary subconscious mind clairvoyance, which is brought about through an altered state of consciousness, such as that resulting from deep meditation, the use of certain drugs, lack of sleep, sensory deprivation, and other cases where the conscious mind of the receiver becomes so quiet that it allows the subconscious mind to come forward and dominate.</u>

Note: *Getting the subconscious mind to dominate is a key component of the Meditative Process- See* **Mind Portal** *Course for complete instructions.*

It is not at all uncommon, for example, for people achieving a relatively deep state of quietude during certain meditation practices to find themselves suddenly swept away from their meditation and propelled into someone else's reality. It may be the reality of someone well known to them or the reality belonging to a total stranger. It all depends on the nature of the sender's subconscious mind networking in place at the time.

INVOLUNTARY PROJECTED CLAIRVOYANCE

Involuntary projected subconscious mind clairvoyance is a clairvoyant phenomenon that occurs most often when we are in a highly emotional state, especially one involving elements of danger. The danger can either be real or imagined.

That is, it can be an actual real life situation or it can be the result of negative thoughts, phobias, psychotic episodes, or even bad dreams or nightmares. Understand that in the world of the mind, the difference between the real and the imagined is sometimes difficult to distinguish.

In either case, whether real or imagined, the emotional, physical, and subconscious mind responses are often the same. We can think of projected involuntary subconscious mind clairvoyance simply as the subconscious mind's cry for help; a sort of psychic international distress call.

The difference between this and a purely telepathic cry for help is that the contactor or projector psychically brings one or more of the recipients to them and forces them to experience everything that they are currently experiencing. In a sense, projected involuntary subconscious mind clairvoyance can accurately be considered the ultimate distress call, where projectors are allowing, although not knowingly, the admittance of another consciousness into their sacrosanct inner world.

THIS IS HOW IT WORKS: When we find ourselves in a life-threatening situation, our conscious mind generates a strong defensive emotional response. This stimulates the subconscious mind to automatically increase the Chi in our aura. If the power in the aura is strong enough, the first requirement for proactive psychic communication is met. Next, the higher mind not only takes advantage of already existing psychic conduits but attempts to create new ones in order to deliver its psychic distress call. Most often, however, those contacted in this manner receive the message in only a telepathic form.

In extremely rare cases, when conditions in the receiver are right, there occurs an exchange of consciousness where the receiver or contactee is actually brought to the projector and experiences first hand the specifics of the projector's circumstances, replete with all of the tactile and sensory experiences occurring at the time.

VOLUNTARY PROJECTED CLAIRVOYANCE

Generally, voluntary subconscious mind clairvoyance is that type of clairvoyance set in motion by those who have acquired a very special level of Chi training. However, there are also certain rare individuals who seem to exhibit this ability naturally. A typical example of voluntary subconscious mind clairvoyance would be that of an advanced mystic calculatingly probing into the present whereabouts and circumstances of a pre-selected subject.

It can either be someone with whom the mystic is familiar, such as a friend or relative, or it may be a person with whom he or she may have had no prior experience at all. It is a matter based solely on the will and needs of the mystic at the time. Because it a deliberate act, voluntary higher mind clairvoyance appears to be much more common than its involuntary counterpart.

This, of course, is not difficult to understand when we consider that the mystic, or receiver of the clairvoyant experience, is also the one who initiates it. Because of this, voluntary clairvoyant experiences are normally devoid of many of the negative qualities, such as anxiety, panic, uncertainty, et cetera, so often associated with involuntary subconscious mind clairvoyant experiences.

That is, of course, unless the seer's contact is ill timed and contact happens to coincide with a particularly perilous or frightening circumstance presently occurring in the life of their subject. Just as we find in involuntary subconscious mind clairvoyance, voluntary subconscious mind clairvoyance encompasses a great deal more than simple telepathy. This is not to say that telepathy is not a useful talent, of course it is; it is just that telepathy and clairvoyance are simply two different types of phenomena.

Unlike telepathy, clairvoyance is not just the transfer of information from the sender to the receiver, but is the actual transfer of supraconscious awareness allowing the mystic or contactor to experience whatever is occurring in the present moment of the subject, replete with all of the emotional bells and whistles that the subject is privy to at the time.

VOLUNTARY SUBCONSCIOUS MIND CLAIRVOYANCE WITH HUMANS

[Step 1] Use the Mind Stilling technique and the Yin chi infusion technique to quiet your conscious mind.

[Step 2] Once your conscious mind has reached a deeply quiet state, mentally picture the person that you wish to experience clairvoyantly. This will automatically create the necessary subconscious mind psychic conduit.

[Step 3] With your conscious mind quiet, use the trigger word "transfer" to initiate the clairvoyant mode in yourself. Your subconscious mind will automatically prepare itself for the coming transfer of consciousness.

[Step 4] Now, when you are ready, pass through your "3rd Eye", and enter the void, traveling through it until you finally pass through the Ajna Vortex of the other person.

Note: *You must not entertain any sense of I-ness. That is, you should not have any conscious thought concerning yourself. If you do, you will have difficulty establishing clairvoyant contact with the subject.*

[Step 5] Maintain the clairvoyant contact as long as you like. When you are ready to break-off contact, will yourself back to your own reality.

SOUL BASED CLAIRVOYANCE

Soul based clairvoyance is arguably the ultimate clairvoyant experience. It has the ability to transcend not only space, as is the case with subconscious mind clairvoyance, but time, as well. That is, soul based clairvoyance can include not only a present circumstance, but can propel us either forward or backward in time.

It is the clairvoyance of the Biblical prophets and gifted seers. In contrast, the subconscious mind, although gifted in many areas, lacks this extraordinary time dimensional elasticity. This is not to say that using the faculties of the subconscious mind without soul involvement we cannot go back in time, we can in a way, but it would be only a limited mock clairvoyant dimensional event made possible by reason of its ability to access the personal memories found in a subject's subconscious mind memory.

Simply, it is not a true clairvoyant returning to the past at all but merely a telepathic memory-based phenomenon. A genuine time-transcending clairvoyant experience must have soul-level origins.

3 DISTINCTIONS BETWEEN SUBCONSCIOUS MIND AND SOUL CLAIRVOYANCE

[1] Subconscious mind-based clairvoyant experiences are restricted to the present.

[2] Any precognitive or antecedent clairvoyant experiences are actually originating at the soul level.

[3] Any information originating at the soul level is pure and accurate. Those coming from or through the subconscious mind are generally not. That is, if the clairvoyant experience is not entirely accurate, then it must have been variously tainted by the subconscious mind and/or the conscious mind in some way.

Voluntary soul-based clairvoyance

Voluntary soul-based clairvoyance is so extraordinary, so awe-inspiringly esoteric, that it is generally experienced only by those deeply initiated in the mysteries of extreme Chi abilities; those who have at their command specific techniques designed to quiet the higher mind to the point where it will not interfere in any way with the transmission of soul-based information.

Without question, the most widely known example of voluntary soul-based clairvoyance would be that demonstrated by Michel de Nostredame [a.k.a. **Nostradamus** 1503-1566] who was able to peer clairvoyantly into both the present and the future, although he is most renowned for the latter. Under the tutelage of his grandfather, he was initiated into the mysteries of the **Jewish Kabbalah**, which formed the basis of all of his subsequent esoteric endeavors.

The use of hallucinogens to aid him in bringing about the necessary quiescence of both his lower and subconscious mind turned out to be a double-edged sword. On the one hand, it did seem to bring him unparalleled success as a clairvoyant seer, but on the other hand, it haphazardly propelled him into a life filled with spontaneous clairvoyant episodes of often frightening and sanity-threatening proportions.

Because of this, we can say that Nostradamus is [or at least should be] the poster-boy for the anti-hallucinogenic drug factions of the mystical world. Nostradamus, however, did not rely solely on hallucinogens. He also employed a number of much safer and arguably more effective concentration techniques to bring about his voluntary soul-based clairvoyance.

One such technique was the Black Bowl or Black Water technique, in which he would stare into a water-filled black bowl, concentrating on the tiny points of light on its surface in order to achieve an extraordinary focus or one-pointedness. Initially, this would be enough to quiet his conscious mind. As his concentration continued, he would penetrate deeper and deeper into the points of light until his subconscious mind fell into a pristine state of quietude.

It was only when he reached this state that he was prepared for the soul-based clairvoyant experiences for which he became so well known. Nostradamus' Black Bowl technique, sans hallucinogens, is an excellent way for a modern mystic to reach a soul-based clairvoyant experience.

It is actually a form of scrying, a method well known among mystics where an object, such as a crystal ball, becomes a sort of movie screen upon which clairvoyant images are projected. In truth, there is nothing at all actually appearing in the black bowl or crystal ball, it is all taking place at either the higher mind or soul level of the seer.

Arguably, it was Nostradamus' ability to achieve soul-based clairvoyance that made his prophecies so relatively accurate. Why relatively accurate? Because, at times, some of his prophecies were apparently distorted through higher and conscious mind interference and were rendered vague and error-ridden. This, coupled with the fact that much of the time he was at a loss to explain what he was actually seeing, made a number of his prophetic accounts rather dubious. Even so, his abilities at soul-based clairvoyance were still quite remarkable and clearly propelled him into a coveted place of mystical prominence.

THE BLACK BOWL TECHNIQUE

[Step 1] Find a quiet place to begin your journey into the future; a place free from noise and distractions.

[Step 2] Seat yourself at a table on which you placed a black bowl filled with clear water. Place a lit candle on the table on the other side of the bowl. Adjust the distance of the candle until you can see points of light reflected on the surface of the water.

[Step 3] Use the Mind Stilling technique and the Yin chi infusion technique to quiet your conscious mind. Do not proceed further until you are absolutely sure that your conscious mind is as quiet as possible.

[Step 4] When you are sure that your conscious mind has reached a deeply quiet state, look down at the surface of the water in the bowl. At first, it will be just a casual looking, noticing without mental comment the various attributes of the water, such as its color, its stillness, and the various points of reflected candlelight on its surface.

[Step 5] When you are ready, begin concentrating on a single point of light. Stare at it until it begins to take on the three-dimensional appearance of solidity. You may blink normally.

[Step 6] When the point of light becomes solid, use the mental trigger word **future**, and begin to penetrate the point of light, traveling deeper and deeper into it until the point of light is all that exists.

[Step 7] Once the trigger word or phrase has been mentally expressed, continue staring at the point of light as it seems to take on a deep and almost infinite character. Continue to do so until your vision contains nothing but the reflected light and everything else in the room is completely obliterated. When this happens, you are primed and ready for the clairvoyant experience. All you have to do now is to wait for it to happen.

IMPORTANT: *Do not have any particular thoughts concerning either the waiting or what you are waiting for. That is, there should be no thoughts such as "now, all I have to do is wait," or "I am now prepared to see the future," or "what's going to happen now?"* **There must not be any thoughts at all present in your mind. If there are thoughts, it means that your conscious mind has become involved and you may have to begin the entire process over again.** *If, however, both your lower and subconscious minds are quiet enough, the soul-based clairvoyant experience should take place, propelling you into the future.*

IMPORTANT: Do not panic when you find that you are suddenly thrust into a different environment; a different reality. Simply observe without mental comment.

[Step 9] When you are ready to return to the present, you can introduce conscious mind thought, such as "well, back to the present," or," it's time to end the session." You may find it very helpful to rub your face with a little water from the bowl.

[Step 10] Now is the time to take notes on your experience. Write down as many details as possible, sorting out the known from the unknown, the identifiable from the unidentifiable, et cetera.

Chapter 5: Precognition, Gazing Into The Past, Present & Future

3 LEVELS OF PRE-COGNITION

There are three levels at which we may psychically receive information concerning the future, each differing both in quality and accuracy.

The first level is the highest and purest of the three. It is the reception of pure, unadorned, information accessed at the ultimate source, the soul. This level of unerring prophecy reveals events which will come to pass without deviation or need for interpretation. This is also the psychic plane of the biblical prophets and the most highly developed mystics.

The second level is that of the subconscious mind. This is the realm of the average psychic, where the originally pristine soul-generated information is received and altered in various degrees, resulting in a precognitive message that is ordinarily a great deal less dependable than that viewed at the soul level. The reason for the decrease in accuracy is that the pure soul-based information received by the subconscious mind is often made impure by associative correspondences existing in the psychic's subconscious mind memory or mind system.

That is, the subconscious mind receives information from the soul and then proceeds, in varying degrees, to superimpose on that information correlative material from one's personal past experiences. For example, suppose that the subconscious mind receives soul-generated information concerning an upcoming financial change in the Real Estate Market.

If there exists in the subconscious mind memory of the receiver any manner of corresponding information or experience concerning real estate, housing, markets, homes moving, childhood homes, family homes, real estate investments, et cetera, in one's past lives, then depending on the depth of that experience, the higher mind may make correlations and wind up misnaming, relocating, or distorting that information in some fashion.

That is, the vision foretelling of a change in the real estate market may, indeed, be correct, however, the particulars of that event may be subtly corrupted, causing the psychic to misname the timing and severity either up or down of the market, and so on. For this reason, many of the predictions coming from psychics seem somewhat anecdotal and unreliable.

The third level at which we access precognitive information is the most common. It is also the basest and arguably the least reliable of the three. It comes to us through the offices of our conscious minds. Understand that the pure and unadulterated information radiating from the soul reaches the conscious mind only after first passing through and being variously altered by the subconscious mind.

The lower mind then takes that already tainted information and proceeds to distort or cover it over even more with large amounts of data coming from its own conscious mind memory system and in accordance with its own particular intellectual processes.

Moreover, if that isn't enough, it also further warps incoming precognitive information by superimposing on that information emotionally-generated images of past correlative events. The fact is that the conscious mind may alter the original precognitive information to the point where it actually becomes oblivious to the very existence of that precognitive information.

That is, the conscious mind veils the precognitive, soul-generated, information so well that it cannot even recognize it as such. Well, believe it or not, the conscious mind still isn't finished. To make matters worse, the conscious mind is often so loud and loquacious that even if it did not produce any distortions at all, the soul generated subconscious mind transmitted precognitive information may not even be heard or received at all, or would, at best, simply degenerate to the form of a sketchy intuitive feeling or a half convincing hunch of unknown origin.

Even so, with all that the conscious mind does to cover or distort what it receives, precognitive information can still come through. Unfortunately, when it does, it arrives in the form of a dream: an often chaotic, yet vaguely familiar scenario riddled with superimposed elements originating from its own memory system.

This is the type of precognitive experience that is often either ignored or greatly misinterpreted. Of course, if an accomplished mystic subjects the experience to proper and rigorous scrutiny, many of the superimposed elements can be eliminated and a somewhat accurate interpretation can often be deduced.

This is what Joseph of biblical fame did when he interpreted the pharaoh's dream of the seven fat cows and the seven lean cows coming up out of the river; he simply saw through all of the superimposed symbolism. Understand that precognition at the conscious mind level, coming in the form of dreams, intuitions, and hunches, is a relatively common event in our lives. To benefit from these experiences, all we have to do is to recognize them as such and learn to decipher them. For beneath all of the cloaking lies the original soul-based precognitive message.

PRE-COGNITIVE EXERCISES

FULL DECK OF CARDS BEGINNERS EXERCISE #1

[Step 1] Quiet your conscious mind by using the Mind Stilling technique and/or the Yin chi infusion technique.

[Step 2] Have your partner mix the deck and place it face down on the table. Then, picking up the first card, he or she will look at it and project the image of the card out through their "3rd Eye".

[Step 3] Travel through your "3rd Eye" and view the image that the sender is projecting, notifying them each time that they project the image of a picture card.

[Step 4] Have your partner continue sending the image of each card until you have identified all of the picture cards in the deck.

FULL DECK EXERCISE #2

[Step 1] Quiet your conscious mind by using the Mind Stilling technique and/or the Yin chi infusion technique.

[Step 2] Have your partner mix the deck and place it face down on the table. Then, have him look at each card one at a time, concentrating on the suit symbol on the card, and project the image of the symbol out through his "3rd Eye".

[Step 3] Travel through your "3rd Eye" until you come across the image that they are sending.

[Step 4] Continue doing this until all of the cards in the deck are used.

FOUR CARD DECK EXERCISE #2

[Step 1] Remove the four aces from the deck.

[Step 2] Quiet your conscious mind by using the Mind Stilling technique and/or the Yin chi infusion technique.

[Step 3] Have your partner mix the four cards and place them face down on the table. Then have him look at each card one at a time, concentrating on the suit symbol, and projecting the image of the symbol out through their "3rd Eye".

[Step 4] Travel through your "3rd Eye" until you come across the image that they are sending. Since the suit symbols are so very different, you should have no difficulty telling them apart.

13 CARD NUMBER EXERCISE

[Step 1] Remove thirteen cards of the same suit [ace-through-king] from the deck.

[Step 2] Quiet your conscious mind by using the Mind Stilling technique and/or the Yin chi infusion technique.

[Step 3] Have your partner mix the cards and place them in a stack face down on the table. Then, have them look at each card one at a time, projecting the image of the number or letter symbol of the card out through his or her "3rd Eye".

[Step 4] Travel through your "3rd Eye", deep into the void, and view the images your partner is projecting, notifying them each time of the name of the card [i.e., a nine, king, ten, etc.]

ZENOR CARD METHOD

[Step 1] Quiet your conscious mind by using the Mind Stilling technique and/or the Yin chi infusion technique.

[Step 2] Have your partner mix the entire Zener deck and place it face down on the table. Then, looking at each card, one at a time, have him or her project the image of the symbol on the card out through their "3rd Eye".

[Step 3] Travel through your "3rd Eye", deep into the void, until you view the image that your partner is projecting. Notify them each time of the identity of the symbol you see.

[Step 4] After you attempt to identify the symbols, the sender will place the card in one of two piles, the correct answer pile or the incorrect answer pile. When you have completed the entire deck, count the cards in the correct pile and record the results.

The law of averages tells us that out of twenty-five cards, getting four or five cards correct can be nothing but pure chance. This being the case, any number of correct answers you make above four or five would clearly be a sign of some degree of telepathic ability.

That having been said, to make only a single pass through the Zener deck would really not affirm very much. Therefore, to get a much more accurate figure, you should run through the entire deck at least four times. This means that your accuracy percentage will be based on a hundred cards rather than only twenty-five. In fact, you should keep a running record of your scores each time you practice. This will indicate, not only your true telepathic ability, but will allow you to see how much improvement you are making.

Chapter 6: Time Travelling With Your Mind

GOING BACK IN TIME

When we first attempt to practice viewing the past it is not uncommon for our memory systems to interfere with our ability to experience the clairvoyant event we are seeking to have. That is, instead of having an actual clairvoyant experience, we find ourselves having nothing more than a vivid subconscious mind memory experience, in which we are simply recalling events from our past lives.

For example, we may believe that we are clairvoyantly traveling back in time to a particular year, but may only be remembering and then viewing events, people, and places that were indelibly recorded in our own higher mind memories during that particular incarnation.

For many, especially, beginners, it is often difficult to tell the difference between a memory experience and an actual antecedent clairvoyant experience. Of course, subconscious mind memory may not be the only cause responsible for having us confuse a clairvoyant experience with a memory experience. Just as we might confuse the viewing of the distant past clairvoyantly with memories recorded in our subconscious mind memory, so might the conscious mind confuse a clairvoyant experience with the viewing of our recent past, those memories recorded in it from our current incarnation.

Here, instead of having a true clairvoyant experience, we may merely be vividly recalling the memories recorded in our conscious mind memory. Of course, telling the difference between viewing our own present-life memories and that of having an actual clairvoyant occurrence would be relatively easy to do. For example, suppose we were experiencing an event that took place in Japan in nineteen hundred and forty-four. We would know immediately whether or not we have any personal information or experience of Japan that occurred at that time.

If we know that do not have any such experience, then what we are witnessing most likely would be an actual antecedent clairvoyant episode. Of course, it can be argued that we may have learned about Japan at some point in our life, in school, at the movies, from books, et cetera, and that the so-called antecedent clairvoyant experience is really only based on that acquired information and nothing more.

Is it possible? Certainly, it is possible. An experienced clairvoyant would be able to recognize the difference immediately. The clues would lay in the differences in not only the quality of the experience but in the presentation of many of the factual elements, as well. For the novice, the distinctions may not be so obvious. Remember that memory, no matter how clearly presented to us, is still just memory.

That is, although it may be more vivid than most, a memory we think is a clairvoyant experience still plays back to us as the recalling of any ordinary memory would. The difference is that in a truly clairvoyant experience, we are actually there, and are experiencing all of the tactile and sensory input associated with being there. We do not have this when simply recalling a memory.

There is yet another way that the lower and higher minds may interfere with the genuine antecedent clairvoyant incident. They may color or distort the various elements involved in the experience in some fashion. For example, we may be having a truly antecedent clairvoyant experience concerning an event with which we did have some present-life prior knowledge, such as the Allies' perspective of the D-day invasion of Europe.

What we have learned about that particular event in school, through reading, in the movies, on television, et cetera, may unduly influence what we are experiencing clairvoyantly by superimposing on it elements in various degrees that may be misleading, such as by superimposing on the clairvoyant experience correlative information previously recorded in our lower and subconscious mind memories.

Here, they may, for example, actually go so far as to project a famous actor or scenes from a movie into the experience. Should this happen, then we will experience nothing but a disjointed clairvoyant collage of the D-day invasion. Would it be an actual antecedent clairvoyant event? Yes, it would, but it would be covered over with non-clairvoyant distortions.

PAST LIFE CLAIRVOYANCE

Understandably, the idea of going back into our past lives is a subject that fascinates many of us. However, past-life clairvoyance is not merely the recalling of events that are recorded in our higher mind memories from our past lives... it is a great deal more.

In past-life clairvoyance, we are actually experiencing a consciousness transition from our own present to our own past, which will include all of the sensory and tactile input that occurred at that specific moment in our past.

We would actually be there, reliving moments in our past incarnations, not merely as a simple observer, but as an actual participant. Naturally, the possibility of us actually being able to do this brings up a very important question: If we could travel back to our past and actually be there, would we then be able to change our past and perhaps alter history in some way?

The answer is both yes and no. In order to understand this answer, we would have to appreciate something of the nature of time and parallel existences. It sounds deep and intriguing doesn't it?

Simply stated: Both time and space exist infinitely within the being of the Eternal. Understand that time and space stretch out in not only an infinite number of directions, but since we are dealing with infinities, we have to accept the idea that there are an infinite number of time-lines, as well as an infinite number of worlds and possibilities existing along those time lines.

When we look at our own lives and our world history, for example, we notice that it is clearly a single time-line moving in a linear manner from the past to the present and from the present onward into the future. However, if we accept the idea of the Eternal as being infinite, we must also accept the idea that everything existing within it must also be infinite.

Because if the Eternal is infinite and if everything is one with the Eternal, then everything must share in that infinity. If this is the case, then we could say that even the most minute part of the Eternal is equal to the whole. It only follows then, that there cannot exist just one time-line within the Eternal's infinite nature. To reject that concept would be contradictory, for it would deny that infinity.

Accordingly, if we accept the proposal that if the Eternal is infinite, truly infinite in all aspects, we would then have to accept the idea that within the Eternal exist an infinite number of planes of existence, as well as an infinite number of time-lines associated with each of them.

Here we have an infinite number of worlds and time-lines that are not only parallel our own but actually must cross our own at an infinite number of points. What this means, in a nutshell, is that, yes, we can go back in time and change our life and influence history, but any changes that take place must occur in a separate and parallel existence along another separate and parallel time-line.

For that reason, we would only be able to visit those changes if we could somehow manage to cross over and remain in that parallel world. Now, when we say no, we cannot alter our past and change history, we mean that it cannot be done because each time-line is immutable.

To make any changes at all, would automatically cause the creation of a new and separate time-line. Of course, when we use the word creation, we are only using it in the figurative sense. This is so because when we are dealing with the infinity of the Eternal, every possible time-line, each replete with infinite minute deviations, must already be in existence.

Therefore, if we seem to change the past when we go back clairvoyantly, it is nothing but an illusion, because all we really would be doing is changing time-lines and worlds, which means that we will not actually change anything in the past of the world in which we presently live.

ADDITIONAL CONSIDERATIONS

Traveling clairvoyantly into our own past requires proper preparation. Do that and the safer and more efficient those journeys into the past will be. Prepare improperly and it would be very much like jumping out of an airplane and trying to figure out how to operate the parachute on the way down. That would not be wise.

To begin, in order to experience past-life clairvoyance, our subconscious mind memory has to be opened, allowing access to information about our past that has been previously been recorded there. Our subconscious mind is our personal link to our past, the doorway to our previous lives.

To bring this "opening" about, our conscious mind must first be made so quiet, so dormant, that all that remains active is our subconscious mind. This can be achieved through proper meditative techniques **(See Mind Portal for Detailed Instructions)**

However, the quieting of our conscious mind is only the first step in the process. Once our conscious mind is brought to a state of absolute stillness, our subconscious mind has to be finessed into bringing our past-life memories forward.

This must be done by a very special thought generated by the subconscious mind, itself. It is really a thought without thought, a product of thinking without thinking. As abstruse as this must sound, it is actually the only way that the subconscious mind has of thinking. Just as our conscious mind comes replete with a mental voice mechanism that allows us to hear the thoughts it produces, our subconscious mind also has a voice.

However, it is one that is so subtle that it produces thoughts that often defy recognition by the majority of us. Hence, we say that it is thinking without thought... thinking without thinking. For us to clairvoyantly access our past lives, we must generate a very special type of thought that will cause our

101

subconscious mind to lay bare the enormous array of past-life memories associated with it. It must be a subconscious mind thought, a thought that the subconscious mind will recognize and accept as its own, otherwise, it will summarily reject our wishes and nothing will be accomplished.

Once our conscious mind is absolutely still, we can use a trigger word or phrase to indicate exactly what we are looking for. Supposing that our subconscious mind accepts the request, what next? How will we know when our higher mind memories are open? The answer is simple: we will know it by the nature of the images that suddenly begin to flash across the screen of our consciousness.

Initially, the images will most likely be sporadic and fleeting, lasting only moments. After that, we may experience an enormous peace during which time we should able to view the memories specified in our trigger phrase. At this point, our subconscious mind memory system behaves and can be accessed in much the same manner as our conscious mind memory system.

That is, we would be able to recall our past life memories as easily as we are able to summon our present life memories. Just as in conscious mind memory recollection, initially only the most salient memories will come to light, memories that were in some particular way significant to us in the past. They may be memories that were ultra-pleasurable and highly rewarding, or memories that were uniquely morose, or grimly traumatic.

We should not be surprised or shocked in any way by what surfaces even if those memories are, in fact, somewhat disturbing. Remember that what we are seeing are just memories.

Of course, being higher mind memories, they are that part of us that we bring back with us each time we reincarnate and are, in some measure responsible for who we are today. Therefore, bearing this in mind, it is clear that our subconscious mind memories are the mystical keys that will unlock and allow us to experience our past lives and uncover the secrets that those lives hold.

ACCESING PAST MEMORIES TECHNIQUE

[Step 1] In a room that is free of distraction, begin a thirty-minute period of meditation **(see Mind Portal for details)** to quiet your lower mind. Note: If necessary, you may have to increase the meditation to sixty minutes or more.

[Step 2] Use the Mind Stilling technique and the Yin chi infusion technique to further quiet your lower mind.

Important: *Do not proceed further until you feel absolutely certain that your conscious mind is as quiet as possible.*

[Step 3] With your eyes closed and your lower mind serene, think the trigger phrase: "my past-life memories." Now, wait.

[Step 4] Once the memories begin to come to you, simply observe them.

Important: *Remain calm and try not to let them overly excite you or your conscious mind may become active and interfere with the flow and clarity of the images.*

Note: *It is important to understand that the events of our past lives are recorded in our subconscious mind memory in chronological order. Even so, they may appear out of sequence,* *possibly even leaping from life-to-life. This is quite natural, especially in the beginning, and is nothing to be concerned about. We must simply observe whatever appears to us.*

[Step 5] To bring yourself out of it, all you have to do is to open your eyes.

Note: *Once we have opened our subconscious mind memory, it has a tendency to stay open, which makes it easier to access past-life memories whenever we choose to do so.*

ONCE THE SUBCONSCIOUS MIND IS OPEN

[Step 1] With your conscious mind quiescent, access your subconscious mind memories and allow them to flow.

[Step 2] When a memory comes to you that you want to investigate further, begin to concentrate on it until the details of that memory make themselves known to you. Naturally, they may seem vague at first, but clarity will come with persistence and practice.

Note: *Remember, viewing memories recorded on your subconscious mind tape is not very different than viewing the memories that you have on your conscious mind tape. Just as the memories you are used to experiencing when you think back on this current life appear in order of prominence, the memories your have on your subconscious mind tape will appear to you in the same manner.*

RECOGNIZING YOUR PERSONAL PAST

Past-life clairvoyance is actually very similar to other more common clairvoyant experiences in that there is an exchange of realities taking place through established subconscious mind psychic conduits.

The main difference, of course, is that instead of being brought into someone else's reality in the present, we are brought into our own reality in the past. That is, the subconscious mind psychic conduit created is self-contained and forms a clairvoyant loop with its own memory system.

Normally, the creation of a subconscious mind clairvoyant loop is volitional, intentionally brought about by those who have the will and knowledge to do so, but there are rare instances when this particular clairvoyant phenomenon is non-volitional, a product of happenstance, in which a person is suddenly and unexpectedly swept into various circumstances of his or her own past lives.

Generally, there are no warning signs to indicate that this event is coming; it simply occurs spontaneously and without warning. Because of this, it is very often a frightening experience for those who find themselves unexpectedly thrust into it. When it happens, often those unfamiliar with this form of clairvoyance believe that they are actually having an astral projection or out-of-body experience. This is understandable since, during the experience, they seem to have the ability to move about at will.

However, instead of being able to move about in ghost-like fashion, as occurs in cases of astral projection, in past-life clairvoyance they are only able to wander about in scenarios bounded by their own past experiences and memories. There is another more typical way to have the sense of free movement during past life clairvoyance episodes.

Paradoxically, it is one actually more common to the casual mystic than to the experienced mystic. This occurs when there is a nexus or connection created between the clairvoyant experience and the memories summoned or triggered by that experience.

In other words, memories, themselves, can and often do give rise to a sense of free movement, even if that movement is merely illusionary.

Confused?

What we are referring to are those types of movements that can occur intentionally and are based on memories that are found in the subconscious mind memory. A sense of free movement can occur, for example, when the clairvoyant finds himself or herself experiencing a former dwelling and by reason of memory can volitionally seem to move about the house, going from room to room and even going outside of the house and onward into town.

Would the clairvoyant actually be moving and in reality going at will wherever he or she wants to? They are not moving at all in the astral projection sense, but in a memory sense we would have to say, yes, they might be said to be moving, for there is still that clairvoyant kineticism that is in place and functioning giving them the sense of voluntary movement. Again, to help make memory-triggered movement clearer, let us suppose that our initial past-life clairvoyant experience has us standing in the kitchen of our sixteenth century Irish country home.

Being there is bound to trigger memories concerning the layout of the house, such as the location of the other rooms. Since the memories of moving about the house are recorded in our higher mind memory, we may find ourself walking from the kitchen to the master bedroom or from the kitchen to the front yard, by reason of the fact that we have done that in the past.

Therefore, what is taking place is a memory-based clairvoyant transfer, giving rise to the notion of free movement. In other words, we can go anywhere we like as long as there are memory paths in place to take us there.

We will find that a single clairvoyant episode will generate an enormous number of such memory paths, which in turn will take us places that will trigger even more memory paths and offer us a greater sense of moving about and seeing places, people, and objects at will from that previous life. As we might imagine, because of these memory paths and our ability to move about on them, it is easy to confuse the experience with astral projection.

Remember, it is important to understand that while we are having an authentic past-life clairvoyant experience, we will not be able to alter or affect the elements of what we are experiencing, such as replacing a sixteenth century outhouse with a modern twenty-first century indoor bathroom.

Remember also, that what we are experiencing are memory-based clairvoyant episodes, founded on events, places, people, objects, and actions that are as they were when they first occurred in our past. If we find that we are able to make any changes, then we can be sure that they will be changes superimposed on our experience through the involvement of our conscious mind.

Beginners have a tendency to do this, often allowing their conscious minds to become actively involved in embellishing their clairvoyant experiences with fanciful elements and concepts. This creates misconceptions and distortions that cloud the truths of the experience, and should be assiduously avoided.

TECHNIQUE FOR EXPERIENCING YOUR PAST

[Step 1] Quiet your conscious mind with 30 minutes of mantra meditation; more if needed.

[Step 2] Use the Mind Stilling technique and the Yin chi infusion technique to further quiet your conscious mind.

[Step 3] With eyes still closed, use the trigger phrase: **my past lives.**

[Step 4] Once the request is made, peer into your "3rd Eye" and travel deep into the void beyond. If your subconscious mind responded correctly, you will be entering the psychic conduit that your subconscious mind has established with itself.

Note: *At first, you may encounter only random images of your past. This is perfectly natural. Remember, you are going back and viewing some of the more salient items or events recorded in your subconscious mind memory. Do not become disturbed if the images come too quickly or they appear somewhat vague.*

[Step 5] When a clear memory comes to you, and you want to investigate it further, simply concentrate on it and a subconscious mind psychic conduit will be established between the you of today and the you of that particular former life. When this happens, you should find yourself suddenly whisked away into that former existence and should be able to re-experience all of the sensory and tactile elements that were occurring at that particular moment in time.

[Step 6] You can remain in that experience as long as you like. To break the loop and return to the present, simply break your concentration by opening your eyes.

WHAT TO LOOK FOR WHILE IN THE PAST

CALENDARS: Are there any calendars on the wall, desk, et cetera, that will tell you the year, month, and day of your experience? If so, in what language is the calendar written? Are there any advertisements on the calendar? Is there anything unusual about the calendar? Are there any notes or special days marked-off on the calendar?

NEWSPAPERS: What is the year, month, and day of that particular issue? What is the headline? What are the leading stories? What is the name of the newspaper and where is it distributed? What language is the newspaper printed in? Are their any ads that will help you in identifying the country, city, and time period that you find yourself in?

LETTERS [personal and business]: To whom are they addressed? Who are they from? What is their content? Are there stamps on the envelopes? If so, what country are they from? Is there a postmark on the envelope that will tell you the city, country, and date? Are the letters sealed with sealing wax? If so, is there anything significant about the design impressed on the wax?

OTHER WRITTEN MATERIAL: Are there parchments, clay tablets, laundry lists, grocery lists, receipts, bank statements, personal or business notes or memos, posters, graffiti, et cetera, to help you identify the place and time of this past life?

HOUSE STYLE: Is there a house or other buildings in your experience? If so, what is the style of architecture? Is the house Tudor style, ranch style, a split-level, apartment building, a temple of some sort, et cetera? Is it constructed of wood, brick, adobe, or other material? How many stories, rooms, et cetera, does it have? Does the building have indoor plumbing? Is it located in an urban, suburban, or country setting? Are there outhouses, barns, sheds, silos, gardens, et cetera, on the property? What are the walls and windows like? Are there numbers on the door indicating an address? Is there anything at all that is strange or unique about the house?

FURNITURE: Are the pieces French traditional, English, Oriental, Scandinavian, et cetera? Are there any unique pieces of furniture? If so, what are they made of and what makes them unique? Are there items of children's furniture? If so, what are the approximate ages of the children that would have such furniture [cribs, bassinets, bunk beds, et cetera.]? What style of bed is found in the master bedroom?

KITCHEN: What type of cooking devices do you see? Is the stove a wood burner, gas operated, or electric? What is the style of the eating utensils? Are they silverware, chopsticks, et cetera? What is the style of the plumbing? Does the kitchen have indoor plumbing? Notice the particular type of water delivery system. Is there a tap or faucet at the sink, a hand-pump, et cetera? Do you see condiments or food in the kitchen? What are they? Is the floor tiled, or made of wood or stone?

PEOPLE: Are the majority of people Caucasian, Black, Oriental, or Indian? What language are they speaking? What hairstyle, hair color, mustaches, beards, et cetera, do the people have? Is there anything unusual about the people in general?

MANNER OF DRESS: What is the nature and style of the dresses, skirts, blouses, hats, suits, et cetera, that you see the people wearing? What period in history are the clothes from? Do the men carry weapons: swords, rifles, handguns, knives, et cetera?

TERRAIN: Do you see mountains, valleys, flatlands, grasslands, wetlands, farmland, rolling hills, or city streets? Are there factories, dykes, walls, totem poles, religious structures, windmills, pyramids, or anything that would help you identify the place and time you are in?

STREET SIGNS: If you are in a city, are there street signs? If so, in what language are the signs written? What do they say? Do they give street names or directions? Are there signs that advertise products or places? Are the signs hand-painted or manufactured?

SHOPS AND STORES: What type of shops and stores do you see? What is the nature of the goods they sell? Is there anything about the goods they sell that can help you identify the place and time period of your experience? Are there any physical design peculiarities that stand out about the shops?

AROUND THE HOUSE: Are there curios or collectables in the house? If so, what are they? What are they made from? Where do the majority of curios seem to come from? How are they stored? Are they in cabinets, on tables, on dressers? What pictures, painting, murals, tapestries, wallpaper, et cetera, do you see? Is there anything about them that might indicate a time period or what country you are in?

LANGUAGE: Are the people speaking German, Russian, Arabic, Japanese, Hindi, Farsi, English, French, Algonquin, Inuit, et cetera?

MECHANICAL DEVICES: Do you see any mechanical devices? What are they designed to do? Are they run by electricity or steam, or are they operated manually? What period in history are they from?

HEATING: Is the house or shop heated by a fireplace, stove, or furnace? Is there anything unusual about the heating apparatus? For example, if there is a fireplace, is there anything odd or outstanding about it, such as an ornamental mantle, special brickwork, inscriptions, et cetera?

WINDOWS: Is there anything odd or special about the windows of the house or building? What do they look like? Are there glass panes in the windows? If so, what is the nature of the glass? Are they clear glass or do they offer a distorted view of the outside? Are they colored or stained? How many panes per window? How many windows are in the room? How many can you see from the outside? Can you tell what period in history their designs are from?

ARTWORK: Are there paintings, murals, or statuary work visible? If so, what is their genre and subject matter? Are the statues made of wood, stone, marble, et cetera? Are there any designs or inscriptions on the walls? Are there wall hangings such as sconces, swords, religious symbols, calligraphy, et cetera?

MIRRORS: What is the design and nature of the mirrors? Are they clear or do they return a somewhat distorted image? What, if any, are the frames like? Are they ornate or plain? If they are ornate, then what details can you discern?

IMPORTANT: *It is vital to understand that if there are mirrors in the house or shop, it may be possible to look into the mirror and actually see what we looked like during that particular incarnation. Even just the memory of having looked into a mirror (or any reflective device for that matter) during an incarnation, can give us a great deal of information concerning our physical appearance, such as our height, weight, approximate age, facial features, and any anomalies we may have had. In short, mirrors are important and their possible existence in our clairvoyant experience should literally be looked into.*

VERIFYING THE EXPERIENCE

It would be fair to assume that whenever we have a clairvoyant experience, we will also have a driving need to know whether or not what we have experienced was real. But how can we verify it?

Where can we go for information, and what should we do first?

The fact that a clairvoyant incident involves someone else's present reality makes it relatively easy to verify. If, for example, the subject is someone that we know, just a phone call will do the trick or, perhaps a visit. Really, just about any standard method of communication will do; phone calls, face-to-face conversation, letters, postcards, telegrams, et cetera.

The point is that all it takes is communication with the other party. That is simple enough. The problems in verification begin when the other party happens to be a total stranger. Here, we have to rely on the information that we received during the clairvoyant experience in order to piece things together.

This makes it important for us to make as many mental notes as we can during the clairvoyant event, covering not only its grosser aspects but its finer, less obvious elements, as well. Obviously, it is important that we become good observers since it will make verification of our experience easier.

After all, it only makes sense that the more information we have, the more information we will have to work with. In the matter of past-life clairvoyance, however, verification may be quite a bit more difficult and time consuming. It may even tax our patience by requiring that we spend enormous amounts of time on the Internet, at the library, in a town hall of records, getting in touch with genealogists, speaking to experts in parapsychology, writing letters of inquiry, sending numerous e-mails, and more.

This is the way of things. Still, it is the sort of investigation that could be fun and ultimately personally rewarding. Unless we happen to have been a well-known historical figure during a particular former incarnation, where gathering information about ourselves is as easy to obtain as looking our name up in an encyclopedia or almanac, we should expect verification of any information concerning us in a former life to take time, often rather large periods of time, so be prepared.

Finally, how much detail we accumulate concerning a former life may not help us verify very much at all, especially if we find that there was a decided lack of record keeping during that particular period. Unfortunately, in such cases, meaningful verification of who we were may even prove to be frustratingly impossible. Even so, we should not take that to mean that our clairvoyant experience was not a genuine occurrence and that we weren't the person that the clairvoyant incident indicated that we were.

ABOUT DREAM STATE PAST RECOGNITION

It is not only possible for our subconscious mind to create a clairvoyant subconscious mind loop and have us experience our past during periods of sleep, but it is in fact, not as rare an occurrence as we might imagine. During a conscious mind dream, any one, or a combination of a number of the elements involved, could find a correlative or equivalent element embedded in the subconscious mind memory.

Should this happen, it could prompt the subconscious mind to create a clairvoyant subconscious mind loop with that memory and the dreamer could suddenly find himself or herself propelled into a past-life clairvoyant experience. Generally, however, when the dreamer awakes, they usually discharge it merely as a vivid dream and summarily dismiss it. Unfortunately, since this form of clairvoyance takes place within the dream state, there is no way to intentionally trigger it.

Even so, when it does happen, the journey into the past is no less impressive or unrealistic than any volitional clairvoyant event. Perhaps the only major difference between the two lies in the ability to intentionally pursue the finer, subtler, details. This means that many of the events in dream-state clairvoyance may be difficult to verify.

Should we suspect that one of our dreams might have actually been a past-life clairvoyant event, we should immediately write down as many of the details as we can remember upon waking. Should we delay in doing so, just as in normal dreams, time will erode the details and clarity of the experience

Chapter 7: Psychometry, Energetic Attachments

PSYCHOMETRY-ENERGETIC ATTACHMENTS

In order to comprehend the mechanics of psychometry properly, certain fundamental particulars associated with the psychometric process must be understood and accepted as axiomatic. Without that acceptance, the entire structure of this explanation would be difficult to understand or appreciate.

One such particular is the enormous natural propensity people have for the creation of higher mind psychic conduits between themselves and the people, animals, plants, and inanimate objects in the world around them. It is through these higher mind psychic conduits that the psychometric information travels, and not by any other means.

The second particular is that the strength of all subconscious mind psychic connections is dependent upon the amount of "attachment" that a person has with another sentient being or inanimate object. Understand the term "attachment" to be all-inclusive.

That is, it is not merely characterized by the love a person has for an object, but can be based on any of our emotions, such as the hate or fear. The third particular is a negative one. That is, inanimate objects do not and cannot absorb, or in some measure retain, the memory of a person having had contact with them. An inanimate object simply does not have the apparatus that would allow it to do that.

UNDERSTANDING PSYCHOMETRY

"The more of an attachment of energy there is in the object, the more of a energetic or psychic conduit will be available"

We have all heard stories of psychics adept at psychometry being brought into mysterious cases as consultants by police and other investigative agencies. There are good reasons for this. As we will see, murders, kidnappings, and other acts of violent antisocial behavior are super-charged with emotional elements that quite readily lend themselves to psychometric investigation.

Understand that where there is emotion, there is attachment, and where there is attachment, there are subconscious mind psychic conduits in place. Therefore, for this first example, we will use a murder scenario, one that is generic in nature and does not make reference to any actual murder committed in the past or present. The murder of our example involves two people; the murderer and his victim.

The site of the murder is a city park. The victim, a middle-aged man, is on his way home one night and decides to travel through the park in order to save time. Walking on a paved path through the park, he is accosted by a glove-clad, knife-wielding, mugger who demands that he turn over all of his money. Frightened by the assailant and his weapon, the man is about to give him his money when a noise off in the distance momentarily causes the mugger to turn away.

The victim seeing an opportunity to escape suddenly bolts down the path. There is a pursuit and the mugger lunges and tackles him to the ground. There is a struggle during which the mugger raises his knife and then plunges it several times into his helpless victim. He steals the man's watch, ring, and money. He buries the victim in a shallow grave beneath a footbridge. Making his way toward the exit, he hears sounds that he believes are a couple of police officers that patrol the park. Not wanting to be caught with the murder weapon, he tosses it into a stand of bushes, and then runs off, eventually leaving the park.

After several days, the victim is reported missing. The police have no clues and are baffled by the man's disappearance. A week later, one of the park's groundskeepers discovers the blood-covered knife and turns it over to the police. However, the knife was examined and no fingerprints were found.

The blood on the knife was analyzed and found to be the same blood type as that of the missing man. The police now have a bloody weapon, but no other clues indicating who are its wielder or victim. At a loss for answers, they call in a psychic, one that they have used with great success in other similar investigations.

At the park, the psychic is given the weapon to hold. She closes her eyes and begins to receive information. She sees the incident from both perspectives; that of the murderer and that of the victim.

What she sees tells not only what happened, but gives her the descriptions of both men. She also sees where the body is buried. The detectives immediately recognize the description of the victim as the man reported missing a few days ago. Following the psychics information, the body is discovered.

Describing the murderer to the police artist, a drawing is created. It is the face of a man that the police have encountered on a number of occasions and so an investigation of the man takes place that eventuates in his arrest and subsequent conviction.

Comments: *How was the consultant able to do it? Did she receive the information from the knife? Many would think so, but no, it wasn't from the knife, it was through the knife. That is, it was made possible by the subconscious mind psychic conduits established with the weapon by both the perpetrator and the victim. The killer had a psychic conduit established because of ownership of and dependence on the knife in his crime and the victim had a subconscious mind psychic conduit established with the knife out of his fear of it.*

The question is: How can a subconscious mind psychic conduit continue to exist intact between someone who is deceased and the weapon that was used to kill him?

The answer lies in the fact that it is the conscious mind that dies, not the subconscious mind. Since the subconscious mind of the victim still functions, the subconscious mind psychic conduit remains in place. Since a subconscious mind psychic conduit always exists between a murderer and his weapon, all a psychic would have to do to retrieve information is establish their own subconscious mind psychic conduit with the weapon.

This will create a link to the subconscious mind of the killer where all the pertinent information is recorded. Of course, it may also create a connection with the subconscious mind of the victim. In either case, the information may very well lead to the solving the crime.

Here, traveling through the established subconscious mind psychic conduit back to the killer would give us information concerning motive, time, place, and other elements that would be pertinent in understanding the event from the killer's perspective. Traveling through the subconscious mind psychic conduit back to the victim would give us information concerning the murder including, but not limited to, a description of the murderer.

EXAMPLE 2

A young man of seventeen was reported missing by his parents. He had left home one night after having an argument with his father. The parents did not suspect foul play, however, a week had passed, and they were worried. He had not attended school during that time and none of his friends claimed to know his whereabouts.

A missing person's report was filed with the police department but their investigation turned up nothing. Desperate to find their son, the parents consulted a woman that they heard was well adept in the use of psychometry. The woman stood in their son's room and asked the parents what object they believed their son loved the most. Both parents, simultaneously, pointed to a high school sweater with a varsity letter on it.

The woman took the sweater and sat down on the bed. She closed her eyes and the images began to come, slower at first, but with more and more rapidity in the following moments. She said she saw a large white house in the country that had a broken white gate. No sooner had she said that that the parents said that their nephew was living in a house like that but that they had spoken to their nephew and he had denied knowing their son's whereabouts.

That evening the parents paid a surprise visit to their nephew and found their son lying on the couch watching television. After a lengthy conversation, all the unresolved issues were settled and everything turned out well.

Comments: *In this example, there was no crime, no weapons, and no evidence. What was there, however, was an object that the missing son had a great amount of attachment for. Again, attachment creates subconscious mind psychic conduits with the object of those attachments. This is what the consultant used to find the boy. Here, all the consultant had to do was create her own higher mind psychic conduit with the sweater. Once this was done, she simply traveled through the boy's established subconscious mind psychic conduit and retrieved the information recorded on his subconscious mind memory.*

EXAMPLE 3

Maria D. was browsing through an antique store when a small, beautifully ornate, wooden music box on a table caught her eye. She opened the lid and it played a lovely tune that she was not familiar with. She had an instant attraction for it and bought it. Later that evening, she sat in her living room with the music box on her lap and examined it more closely.

She opened the lid and the music began to play. Resting her hands on the box, she closed her eyes and lay back on the sofa to listen. Suddenly, random images began flashing across her mind; images of another time, another place. She saw images of the music box sitting on a dressing table in someone else's home. She also witnessed random images of people dressed in clothes from another era and places that she didn't recognize.

At first, she thought that it was nothing more than her imagination, but she soon began to realize that, perhaps, it was more; much more. When she opened her eyes, the images disappeared. She spent most of the night thinking about the images. The next morning, filled with curiosity, she went back to the antique store and questioned the proprietor about the history of the music box. He explained to her that the music box came from the estate of a woman who had died some six months prior, at nearly one hundred years of age.

He went on to explain that, until just recently, the music box had been in storage since that time. One of the visions that Lisa had seen was of a silver comb and brush set with the initials P. T. R. ornately inscribed on the back of the brush. She questioned him about it. The man was astonished by her questions. He told her that he would be right back and excused himself.

He went into a back room and returned moments later holding a small white cardboard box tied with white string. He placed the box on the counter and untied the string. He opened the box and removed the packing paper revealing a silver comb and brush set with the initials P. T. R. inscribed on the back of the brush.

Maria was absolutely astounded. The man went on to explain that the initials P. T. R. stood for Patrice Thelma Reddenberg and that the music box, comb, and brush were hers. He also went on to explain that, from what he could understand, the music box was her most prized possession. Both Maria and the owner of the antique store were amazed at how Lisa had come into her knowledge of the comb and brush.

Comments: *In this example Maria, although not having had a psychic experience of this magnitude before, had formed an instant attachment for the music box. This resulted in the establishment of a subconscious mind psychic between them. Since the former owner, Miss Reddenberg, had died only six months prior, she apparently had not reached total separation. Since she had a great attachment for the music box, the higher mind psychic conduit she had established with the music box was still in place and operational. Here, the music box acted as a connector between Maria's subconscious mind psychic conduit and that of Miss Reddenberg. That connection had Maria receiving images from the deceased's higher mind memory and among them were the images of the silver comb and brush set.*

PROXIMAL PSYCHOMETRY

Proximal Psychometry Subconscious mind Psychic Conduits occur automatically whenever we touch an object or are close enough to an object, enough for our auras to touch it.

They occur whenever we hold, touch, or stand near to a person or object.

When we do, the aura of the person or object is brought into direct contact with our own aura. When this happens, our subconscious mind becomes defensive and begins to probe for answers as to nature of the object that entered its precincts. The subconscious mind establishes a psychic conduit with the object and then begins a process of information retrieval, in which it seeks out and uses any and all psychic conduits that have been established with it. This is the Proximal Psychometry process.

AN EXERCISE TO TRY

[Step 1] Choose an object through which you would like to retrieve information. It could be any object, of course, but it would be a great deal more interesting to choose an object that can offer some insight into a past historical event or one associated with a person known to you that will allow you to verify the information you receive.

[Step 2] Quiet your conscious mind using the Mind Stilling Technique and the Yin chi infusion technique.

[Step 3] Pick up the object and hold it lightly in your hands. Then, close your eyes and relax a moment. With your eyes still closed, peer deep into "3rd Eye" [located in the center of your forehead between your eyebrows]. Have the sense of traveling deep, deep, deep within the void. Whatever information your subconscious mind will receive will be presented to you there.

TELEPSYCHOMETRY

Subconscious mind psychic conduits are established constantly with objects at distances extending well beyond the precincts of a person's aura. In fact, the object could be anywhere in the world or even beyond it. Here, time and distance are of little consequence, because those subconscious mind psychic conduits are established whenever we think of an object.

Remember, the moment a subconscious mind psychic conduit is established with an object, an energy transfer occurs and the subconscious mind begins an information retrieval process. As is the case with proximal psychometry, the subconscious mind will automatically seek out all psychic conduits that have been established with that object by other people. This sets up and fulfills the fundament requirements necessary for telepsychometry.

AN EXERCISE IN TELEPSYCHOMETRY

[Step 1] As in prior exercises, choose an object that you want to use to retrieve information: an object that can give you some insight into a past historical event, or an object associated with a particular person that will allow you to verify any of the information that you receive.

[Step 2] Quiet your conscious mind using the Mind Stilling Technique and the Yin chi infusion technique.

[Step 3] Remember, the object you choose for this exercise may be located anywhere in the world. A photograph of the object would, of course, be helpful, but if none are available, then a detailed description of the object would have to serve. If you are using a photograph, you must stare at it until you are able to close your eyes and see the image of the object in your mind's eye. Once the image is burned in as a negative image, send the Chi out in a circular pattern. Having the information come back like a boomerang effect.

[Step 4] Now, with your eyes still closed, peer deep into the "3rd Eye" [located in the center of your forehead between your eyebrows]. Have the sense of traveling deep within the void. Whatever information or images your subconscious mind receives will be presented to you there.

MOLECULAR PSYCHOKINESIS

Molecular psychokinesis is an extremely interesting phenomenon that takes place whenever Chi is either injected into, or withdrawn from, an inanimate object. The target of the augmentation or reduction of Chi is the object itself and not its aura.

The use of molecular psychokinetic procedures actually results in tangible, often obvious, changes in the target object's physical characteristics. For example, when Chi is injected into a metal, such as brass, the brass becomes soft and pliable at the point of energetic entry.

Conversely, if Chi is withdrawn from a piece of brass, then the brass becomes brittle and readily snapped under light to moderate physical stress. This is true with all metals [silver, iron, steel, et cetera], as well as objects made of sundry other materials, including, but not limited to plastics, glass, et cetera.

Chapter 8: Manipulating Energy, Protecting & Healing

CHI INFUSION

Science tells us that there is molecular motion occurring constantly in all animate and inanimate things. However, since we are currently dealing with inanimate objects, we will address only them for now, and leave our discussion of animate objects for the section on Physiological Psychokinesis.

What is molecular motion? For simplicity, we can think of molecular motion as a vibration peculiar to a particular object or material at the molecular level. Since all inanimate objects are composed of molecules, they all have a natural vibration.

Each vibration is peculiar to a particular object. In Molecular Psychokinesis we influence inanimate objects by altering their molecular activity. There are several factors that affect the vibration of molecules in inanimate objects: temperature, pressure, et cetera.

For us, the most important factor would be that of temperature.

The rule is: *As the temperature of a material increases, there is a corresponding increase in its molecular activity or vibration. Conversely, the same is also true: As the temperature of a material decreases, so decreases its molecular vibration.*

Increases or decreases in molecular activity create changes in the nature of the material. For example, if we heated a piece of plastic and the temperature rose high enough, the plastic would melt. The same example, of course, could be applied to metals. When heat is applied to an object, the energy levels of the molecules that comprise that object are increased, which produces physical changes.

Suddenly, the object is not quite what it was. Chi is energy. When it is injected into an object, the added energy increases the object's molecular motion. This augmentation of molecular activity creates heat, which only further amplifies its activity.

Unless left alone to cool and regain its natural vibration, a sort of molecular heat-producing chain reaction is created, eventually leading to physical changes when the energy levels are high enough. The changes that occur, of course, depend on the nature of the materials that make up the object receiving the added energy. When we work with Molecular Psychokinetic energetic infusion, we must take this factor into consideration.

PULLING CHI OUT OF SOMEONE

All sentient life forms require chi or energy in order to live, this is axiomatic. When chi is plentiful all of a sentient entity's energy requirements are met and, barring disease or injury, all of it cells and organs are able to function properly. However, should an entity suffer a marked decrease in chi that brings its energy levels low enough, there will be a corresponding decrease in the ability of its organs to function correctly.

If this energetic deficit is sustained long enough, the body will undergo a subconscious mind-orchestrated redistribution of whatever energy it does have available to it. That is, the subconscious mind creates a new set of priorities for the allocation of the available energy in order to preserve life. When energy levels become low enough, for example, the subconscious mind of a plant or animal will shut down those organs and functions, at least temporarily, that it deems unnecessary for immediate survival.

It will, for instance, in the case of a person, assure the necessary energetic requirements of the heart and lungs by shunting chi to it from other parts of the body, such as the kidneys, reproductive system, digestive system, etc. Once the heart and lungs' energy requirements are met, it will then assure the proper functioning of the other essential organs by similarly reducing the energy it supplies what it considers non-essential elements of the body, such as the cerebral cortex portion of the brain.

In fact, if the chi supply is at dangerously low levels, the subconscious mind may terminate a pregnancy or may actually reduce the energy supplied to the brain to the point where it will intentionally induce coma in order to conserve the body's chi, and thus to preserve life. Bearing the above in mind, clearly, someone well-versed in the techniques of physiological psychokinesis can cause great injury to the body of another sentient life form by withdrawing from that entity enough chi to initiate a breaking down of their organ functions.

One adept in proper physiological psychokinetic technique has a choice. He or she can withdraw chi from the aura or actually target individual organs for direct disruption. Withdrawing chi from the aura is essentially a generic way to disrupt the energy of an organism.

When the energetic level of the aura becomes low enough, the entity's subconscious mind of the life form will go through the reorganization of its energy priority list on its own and, in effect, determine the results itself.

A person adept at the practice physiological psychokinesis looking to harm another life form would most likely prefer to target specific organs. This requires that the organ be isolated in the mind of the practitioner and a subconscious mind psychic conduit be established with the target organ to the exclusion of everything else. When the properly executed, the effect is quite remarkable and the consequences, of course, quite perilous. Therefore, the physiological psychokinetic withdrawal of chi is something that is not to be practiced indiscriminately or capriciously. We must be guided by good moral judgment, remaining as harmless and blameless in all things as much as possible.

MANIPULATING SOMEONE'S CHI

Regardless of the seeming justification for feelings of vindictiveness the manipulator may have toward their victim, all malice must be eliminated, for such thoughts are products of conscious mind processes and will only serve to pollute the outcome. Therefore, the first order of business must be to quiet the conscious mind to the point where the subconscious mind can be readily accessed.

To do this properly a period of meditation is called for. Of course, when such feelings are removed, there is the possibility that the manipulator may change their mind about taking such a malevolent action. If this should happen, then it is just as well, for we should, whenever possible, be harmless and blameless in our dealings with each other. Still, if the manipulation is to proceed from this point, since the conscious mind is no longer participating in the action, it may seem as as though the manipulation is taking place in an almost matter-of-fact way, devoid of strong emotional attachment.

In fact, to the casual observer, it would even seem to be a cold, passionless, and impersonal process. Nevertheless, this is the way it has to been done. We could say that it is the nature of the beast, and to do it with all of the fervor and passion often depicted in books and movies would actually be self-defeating and ultimately lead to unsatisfactory results.

YOU MUST HAVE AN OPEN GATE TO MANIPULATE WITH CHI

The second factor necessary to establish the manipulation involves the establishment of an open and functioning subconscious mind psychic conduit between the manipulator and the recipient.

This provides the means with which to set up and embed the malediction firmly in the subconscious mind of the recipient. Because subconscious mind psychic conduits established between sentient beings are gated, we must take care not to cause the recipient to close their gate.

If they do, we will not be able to complete the manipulation. Therefore, we must introduce the manipulation in a very subtle, almost benign, way. The process may even require the use of a "gate-opener" in order to be successful.

The reason for this is, there is most likely enmity existing between the manipulator and the recipient, and a functioning open-gated psychic conduit would generally not exist, unless the manipulator and the person being manipulated have not had prior negative dealings together, which is so in cases where a person wishing to manipulate another person seeks a third person, generally unknown to the victim, to perform the manipulation.

Here, since the third person does not harbor strong negative feelings towardthe victim, open-gated psychic conduits would be relative easy to establish and maintain. Another method of assuring that an open-gated subconscious mind psychic conduit is established with a victim is indirect.

That is, by using any open-gated conduits they have already existing between themselves and another person, such as a close friend or relative. Here, that third person becomes the unknowing dupe of the process.

In such a case, it is helpful if the manipulator is on friendly terms with that person, or, at the very least, that no enmity exists between them. Someone adept at manipulating in this fashion would be able to manipulate anyone that they want, simply by sending their malevolent transmissions through one, two, or a series of connected acquaintances of their victim.

Yet another method of reaching a victim through already established open-gated subconscious mind psychic conduits, is to use the working conduits that the recipient has established with inanimate objects, such as their favorite chair, coat, car, et cetera. Here, of course, the conduit established between the manipulator and the object would be ungated and readily created.

117

So, also, would be the conduit existing between the object and the victim. Even so, the manipulation must be delivered in a subtle manner, for the subconscious mind of the victim may still act defensively and remove, at least temporarily, the conduit established between themselves and the object.

Finally, there is this... the manipulator may use parts of the victim's person, such as hair, fingernail clippings, etc. This, of course, is a preferred method in some voodoo practices. This is because a subconscious mind psychic conduit is very easy to establish with their victim since the object, such as pieces of their hair will be readily recognized and accepted by the higher mind of the subject.

Remember, when a recipient's gate is closed, there will be no viable, invocable manipulation possible. Any of the methods mentioned above, if properly performed, should eliminate the problem.

EMOTIONS AND ENERGY

Did you know that we curse or bless people all of the time without realizing it? It's true. Whenever we think of someone we establish subconscious mind connections with them through which energy and information passes.

If, for example, we cede energy to them while the subconscious mind psychic conduit is in place and operational, they are being "blessed" with extra energy and we, losing energy, are actually cursing ourselves, unless we are using a circular method (always recommended) of chi. If, on the other hand, we are lower in energy than they are, energy will flow from them to us. Here, they are being cursed and we are being blessed. (This would only be correct if the Chi is being sent out in a linear fashion. If you circle the chi out, it will always come back, thus eliminating the loss of chi.)

Ordinarily, the energy exchanged in this fashion is briefly delivered or taken, however, if we think about a person frequently, or worse, if we mentally fixate on a person, then this could mean that there may be a flow of energy in one direction or another almost constantly.

This may be all right with someone that we love but what about those people that we have developed a hatred for?

Should we care about their welfare? Well, how would we feel if the person that we hate actually benefits from our fixation on them?

Worse, what if our fixation actually turns around and hurts us?

This is what happens when the focus of our lives revolves around hatred. We are leaving ourselves open to possible harm and are, in essence, cursing ourselves. Therefore, we should let go of feelings of hatred toward others, even our worst enemies, and free ourselves from the possibility that our very own hatreds could not only turn around and cause us immeasurable damage but actually benefit the people we hate.

Note: *We have personal experience with those that use their chi in a way to hate others. In all cases those with the hate tend to have the energy circle back to them and affect them in a very negative way. The saying* **"What goes around, comes around",** *is a perfect analogy in this case.*

HYPNOTIC MANIPULATION & CONTROL

The fact that the subconscious mind exercises an enormous influence over the conscious mind makes it easy to understand that by instilling in the subconscious mind certain ideas, certain scenarios, one well-versed in the art of HYPNOTIC INFLUENCE & CONTROL has the power to create everything from minor illusory disturbances to full scale phobias, from neurotic anomalies to psychotic episodes of devastating proportions and more in his or her victim. The possibilities are really only limited by the HYPNOTIC CONTROLLER'S prowess and individual imagination.

For more information See- Mind Force Hypnosis

A skilled HYPNOTIC CONTROLLER can, for example, create higher mind memories of situations and events that have never taken place, artificial reminiscences that are so powerful and disturbing that they may completely over-shadow their victim's conscious mind reality and create innumerable mental difficulties for them. A skilled HYPNOTIC CONTROLLER can, for instance, place in their subject's subconscious mind memory an experience, such as that of being locked in a very small, dark, area for a long period of time. This may be done to supply the subject's conscious mind with all of the elements necessary to induce claustrophobic reactions in the subject's life. Certainly, the creation of phobias would be a relatively easy process for a talented HYPNOTIC CONTROLLER.

A HYPNOTIC CONTROLLER can also project into the subconscious mind memory of their subject images of great abuse at the hands of a person close to them and by so doing create for their victim an instant dislike or even hatred for that person.

Another rather interesting use of HYPNOTIC MANIPULATION & CONTROL is to create, imaginary, mind-based diseases and pain in their subject. Since the subconscious mind is responsible for the welfare and protection of the body, the creation and installation of psychosomatic symptoms in a person targeted is not difficult to do.

Most of us are well aware that the conscious mind is highly suggestive, readily influenced by events and objects we come into contact with daily; however, we are also being influenced by things and events that exist on the inside, within the confines of our own conscious mind and its associative memories.

The lower mind becomes even more receptive to suggestion when a person's own subconscious mind is the culprit doing the influencing.

Why? It is because there is no place for the conscious mind to run, no shelter from the storm of ideas and images presented to it by the subconscious mind.

Since the elements necessary to produce HYPNOTIC MANIPULATION & CONTROL are installed in the subconscious mind of the victim, the victim's own subconscious mind will complete the task and any further involvement a HYPNOTIC CONTROLLER may want to have with them would generally be unnecessary.

119

That is, once the seed of the HYPNOTIC MANIPULATION & CONTROL is planted firmly in the subconscious mind of the victim, an experienced HYPNOTIC CONTROLLER will simply let nature take its course.

HOW TO MANIPULATE WITH CHI

[Step 1] Think of the person that you want to manipulate. This will automatically establish the subconscious mind psychic conduit between you. A photograph of the person would be helpful.

[Step 2] A good rapport between you and the receiver must then be established. To do this you must make every effort to assure that your initial telepathic contact is as benign and non-aggressive as possible, even though your intentions may not be so benign.

[Step 3] You must have a clear image of just what it is that you want to transmit. Make sure that you do not confuse the receiver with picture-words that appear in your mind that have nothing to do with the message that you want them to receive. It could be a nightmarish scene or you could place images in their mind that you know cater to their particular fears. From the positive side, you could do it as a win/win business deal that will come to fruition.

[Step 4] Once you have the image clearly in your mind's eye, enter the void through your "3rd Eye" and place the image there. Then, project it deep into the void until you feel a subtle release of pressure. When this happens, the psychological manipulation has begun. You can also create an image loop, that you allow them to trigger whenever they think of a certain thing (their spouse, children, job, friends, etc)

Chapter 9: Psychic Self-Defense, Protecting The Energy Body

PSYCHIC SELF-DEFENSE

We are all subjected to psychic influences throughout our lives. Some of them are beneficial and help us in various ways to survive and flourish. Others affect us in negatively by sapping our strength, restricting our movements, creating fear, destroying our health, disturbing our peace of mind, and subtly covering over the deeper and most basic truths concerning ourselves and our personal relationship with the world around us. Unfortunately, this is, despite our liking or disliking, an intricate component of the world within which we all live.

Ironically, we take self-defense lessons, buy handguns, hire body guards, install burglar alarm systems in our vehicles and homes, carry pepper spray, build fences, and do ten thousand other things to protect ourselves, all in the possibility that the day may come when our physical safety might be compromised.

Yes, we do these things and more, and yet, many of us, not realizing that we are variously subjected to negative psychic influences that cause, or have the potential to cause us enormous harm, do nothing whatsoever to protect ourselves against them. Experience and research has told us that there are definite steps that we can take to defend ourselves against this natural phenomenon. All we have to do is to become aware of their existence and take the necessary action when they actually do occur.

ENERGY VAMPIRES

Clearly, there are exchanges of chi taking place in our lives all the time; exchanges between us and both the inanimate and animate objects in our environment. Most of them are not at all harmful to us, some are actually beneficial. The rest, however, whether voluntary or involuntary, are detrimental to our well-being.

Of all the types of psychic attack we may encounter in our daily lives, by far the most common is that inflicted on us by [for lack of a better expression] the "energy vampire." They seem to be all around us... human vampires, animal vampires, and even plant vampires, any and all of which can drain us of our precious energy.

We know that whenever we think of a person, place, or thing, a subconscious mind psychic conduit is automatically created through which energetic energy passes, from the greater to the lesser; from the surplus to the deficit. If we have the energetic deficiency, then we become the energetic vampires and receive energy, which is not necessarily a bad thing.

However, if there is a deficiency of chi in a person, animal, plant, place, or thing, with which we have an open-gated subconscious mind psychic conduit established, that is not good for then they can, and often do, silently draw energy from us. This can leave us feeling drained and tired as our day progresses.

Even worse, it can actually deplete us of energy to the point where we become more susceptible to disease and emotional problems. Bearing this in mind, we must now address the subject in a little more depth, including how we can defend ourselves against them.

HUMAN CHI VAMPIRES

When it comes to energetic vampirism, human beings are, by nature, one of the greatest causes of our daily energy depletion. However, in all fairness, it is not necessarily something that they do intentionally. It all depends on the state of their energy levels and requirements at any given time. Clearly, people not only occupy our thoughts frequently throughout the course of our day, but we also make contact with them at work, shopping, at play, and of course, at home.

They even play both the central and supporting characters of our dreams. It seems, awake or asleep, there simply is no way for us to avoid them. We know when we are in the presence of an energy vampire by the feeling of depletion we experience when we are with them; they just tire us out.

Certainly, each of us has had this experience this at one time or another. Fortunately, thanks to our subconscious mind, we have natural, innate, defenses in place to help us guard our energy resources against these energetic predators.

Fortunately, our subconscious mind, the guardian of our body and its resources, knows when we are losing energy to others and immediately begins a process to rectify the situation. One of the things it does is send urgent messages to our conscious mind as to the cause and nature of the energy drain.

The problem is that our conscious mind, generally being loud and preoccupied much of the time, cannot understand the "letter of the message," only the sense of it. This "sense of the message" frequently creates in us an instant dislike for the person depleting us and we find ourselves looking to separate from them as soon as possible.

In fact, we may actually develop such a defensive dislike for some people that we try to avoid all future contact with them. We must understand that this type of response has nothing to do with personalities, political views, religious affiliations, eating habits, sexual orientations, or personal biases, it is purely self-defensive.

We should bear in mind that energetic vampires come in all sizes and shapes and have different energy needs depending on what happens to be occurring in their lives at the time. The ill, for example, are generally low in chi and are therefore in great need of more in order to quicken their recovery. This places them in the unenviable but necessary position of having to draw chi from all of those who come into contact with them.

122

This is why many people are generally uncomfortable visiting the sick, and why, when they stay too long, become very edgy and out of sorts, and look to leave the moment the opportunity presents itself. Visiting someone in the hospital typifies this experience.

Yes, we may look forward to the visit, but once we are at the patient's bedside, we find ourselves not wanting to stay too long. We may even become clock-watchers, secretly counting down the seconds for visiting hours to be over. The feeling of edginess and wanting to leave that we experience is nothing more than the product of our subconscious mind self-defenses at work.

There is more to energetic vampirism than just being drained when we are in the physical presence of a energetic predator. If we happen to occupy the thoughts of someone during the course of the day, a natural subconscious mind psychic conduit is temporarily established between us. If this person happens to be low in chi, we will lose energy also. It is a sort of tele-energetic vampirism in which we are subtly being relieved of our energy from a distance.

If a person or group of people well-versed in the process of voluntary energy vampirism selects us as the object of their malevolent fixation, we may find ourselves in a potentially dangerous position. The question is: How can we determine when we are being targeted in this way? Certainly, a sense of fatigue would be a common symptom of such an attack, but it is not enough to make a determination.

The inability to move after waking up from a nap is also a frequent indicator of this sort of volitional energetic vampirism, one that can be very unsettling to those who fall victim to it. It feels as if we are being held down or temporarily paralyzed.

The reason that this phenomena occurs is that while we sleep, there was such a drain of chi from us that our muscles temporarily lack the necessary energy to respond. However, once our subconscious mind recognizes the problem and directs a fresh supply of chi to the muscles, we are released from that paralysis and everything soon normalizes.

Yet another common symptom of energetic vampirism is a sudden and seemingly inexplicable sense of disorientation. One moment we seem fine and the next moment we feel dizzy and may even feel as if we are going to faint. Certainly, this is not to say that it couldn't be caused by a physiological condition, such as those that might result from a lack of adequate food or sleep; it could be. Still, we shouldn't dismiss the idea that it may be the result of a sudden loss of chi brought about either intentionally or unintentionally, by an outside agent.

If you are sensitive enough, you can usually feel the chi being pulled or drained from your body. This chi usually is drained from the joint areas of the body. Pay attention next time you around one of these vampires, and see if you can feel the chi being "sucked" out of your body.

We must understand that whether we are being drained of chi intentionally or unintentionally, we are still being drained, and are in some degree, potentially at risk. Of course, if the energy drain is minor, then the danger is minor and is therefore nothing to become overly troubled about. However, if the energy drain is prolonged or suddenly massive, then we may be in great peril, and should address it defensively.

CHI VAMPIRES IN BUSINESS

In business, energetic vampirism is a factor that should be carefully considered. When we are low in chi, for example, we can be sure that our client's subconscious mind is aware of it. This awareness propels their subconscious mind into a defense mode in order to prevent us from draining energy from them. When this happens, the client's subconscious mind closes its psychic gate and whatever rapport we want to establish, or has been established with them, will be lost. And so, in all probability, so will be the sale or deal.

Let us take a moment to imagine what it might be like to be on the receiving end of a salesperson's pitch who happens to be an energy vampire. Imagine what it would be like if, during the conversation, our subconscious mind is frantically trying to advise our conscious mind that we are under attack, and we must end the meeting as soon as possible.

If we can imagine this scenario, then it is easy to know why so many of our attempts to transact business in the past, under similar circumstances, may have turned out so unrewarding. This is something to consider.

Of course, if we, ourselves, happen to be energy vampires, the question would then be why would we need self-defense? Well, we wouldn't, if we didn't care about making that deal or selling that product.

However, if we do care and want to succeed in that business transaction, then we may want to consider raising our energy levels to the point where we have such a large quantity of chi available to us that we actually become energy donors.

If we do that, it will mean that the person that we are trying to do business with will be receiving really nice euphoric and blissful chi from us throughout the course of our meeting and his or her subconscious mind will happily keep the gate open at their end of the subconscious mind psychic conduit. This will cause their higher mind to transmit to their conscious mind the sense that something extremely good is taking place, something very beneficial. This will create a special bond, a workable rapport, with the client and that means success. This is psychic self-defense too.

Many business people's problems are not in the product or in how they dress, but merely a question of energy exchanges and conscious mind impressions based on subconscious mind defense mechanisms. When you "donate" chi to someone that makes them feel really good, you get the obvious good feedback and are succesful in what you do. When you emit stagnent or stale chi, the person feels that too, and want to get as far away and as fast as they can from you.

DEFENSE AGAINST CHI VAMPIRES

Fortunately for all of us, nature has supplied us with some extraordinary natural defenses against the human energetic vampire, foremost of which is the innate ability that our subconscious minds possess to close the gate at our end of any unwanted or potentially dangerous subconscious mind psychic conduit, either in place or attempted to be established with us. This, of course, often puts an end to the possibility of human-based energy drains automatically.

The reason we say "often" is because there are times when subconscious mind psychic conduits are established by knowledgeable occultists; people who know the ins and outs of the conduit process and are skilled enough to be able to circumvent this defense, at least temporarily.

They may have learned how to reach their victims indirectly by establishing subconscious mind psychic conduits with people that the victim knows and has open-gated subconscious mind psychic conduits in place with, such as those normally existing between friends and relatives.

Since the people chosen to act as intermediaries are not generally being drained of energy themselves, their gates often remain open and tender the energetic vampire virtually uninterrupted access to their intended victim's energetic stores. That is, until the victim's subconscious mind realizes what is taking place and closes its psychic gates to that particular friend or relative.

Whether our friends, relations, or for that matter, anyone we know, are energetic vampires, or the unwitting agents of energetic vampires, closing our psychic gates to them can strain or even destroy relationships by replacing a once warm rapport with an uncomfortable sense of distance.

Unfortunately, there is no hiding this distancing when it occurs and we can expect some questioning comments from them about it. Of course, the reason for the sense of distancing may be something else entirely. It could be that the person in question may have defensively closed his or her psychic gates to us, in which case we, ourselves, may be the energetic vampire or the unwitting agent of one.

Clearly, a natural gate-closing defense is almost certainly a relationship destroyer, decimating friendships, business relationships, and even marriages. In fact, as to marriages, one factor that should be taken into consideration when they begin to fall apart is the possibility that one of the partners may be so constantly low in chi that there has a continuous drain of energy on the other partner. This causes them to defensively close the gate at their end of the psychic conduit and emotionally draw away.

This distancing, unless caught in time and reversed, is tantamount to the beginning of the end. It is a cataclysmic energetic snowballing effect that places such enormous strains on a marriage that divorce at some point in time is inevitable.

In the very least, it is something that marriage counselors should learn to recognize and address. Even so, when one partner is constantly draining the other of energy, merely talking out problems is not going to save the marriage. In time, unless the siphoning stops, dissolution of the marriage will be the only way that the energetic vampire's victim has of surviving.

In cases like this, the only way a marriage can be saved is to place the partner who is chronically low in chi on a specific regimen designed to raise their energy to sufficient levels and, consequently, remove the need for them to draw so excessively on their partner's energetic stores. Unfortunately, not until then will the psychic gates reopen and the distancing end.

When you are a competent Chi Power Practitioner, it is very easy to pump up your spouse to give them the extra energy that they need to live life to the fullest. Keep in mind that every time you engage in sexual intercourse with your spouse, you are transfering a part of your energy to them during the love making process. The more times you do this, the closer you will become to your spouse.

125

You can share your chi with all members of your family, by circulating out towards them. Make a habit of filling your house up with good euphoric blissful chi and you will noticy the harmony in your home at an all time high.

ANIMAL VAMPIRES

Humans are not the only energy vampires we come across on a daily basis - animals can be and often are, energy vampires, too. Yes, even that cute and cuddly puppy or kitten can be a little energy Dracula nestling on our lap and quietly draining us of strength.

But don't panic, it is something that takes place all the time in the animal kingdom and is not necessarily a bad thing. It may, in fact, be beneficial. Those of us who have pets are certainly aware of how often they nap during the course of a single day. Cats, for example, take on the average, nearly seventy separate naps a day. Dogs, take a large number of naps, also. The reason for this is that their energy reservoirs are relatively small, which requires them to take frequent naps in order to conserve and restore their life force levels.

Normally, animals, especially adult animals, remain aloof from each other, not only because of practical physical self-defense and pecking order considerations, but also because they are not very willing to cede energy over to each other. Animals have relatively quiet lower minds, which makes them very sensitive to energy fields and energetic exchanges.

This sensitivity generally has them seeking the company of those that can give them energy, rather than those that quietly siphon it from them. Humans, of course, have enormous quantities of chi compared to other members of the animal kingdom. This places us in the unique position of being great sources of chi for them. When an animal is fortunate enough to be a pet, we can be sure that it will take full advantage of our chi supply at each and every available opportunity.

When an animal trusts us, as our pets normally do, open-gated subconscious mind psychic conduits are created between us through which a small quantity of energy continuously flows to them. Naturally, they will take as much as they can get. They will also try to take chi from us by bathing in our chi-rich auras as often as they can. For them, our auras are the place to be. Of course, besides liking to lie down next to us, they also like to be petted.

Petting allows for a temporary merging of auras, which also allows these little vampire-pets to drain off part of our chi. However, their need for chi does not mean that our pets do not love us or give us something in return, of course they do. The fact is that it is a totally symbiotic relationship, meaning that we both benefit from the relationship. They receive a small portion of our energy and we acquire, not only feelings of love and companionship from them, but something else, something really quite remarkable.

We get to have a living, loving, non-addictive, mild sedative at our beck and call. Believe it or not, there are times when we actually have too much chi in our auras. This can actually be harmful to the body, by causing it to become over-active and to over-function. This is not at all advantageous to our well-being and the subconscious mind knows it. To remedy this situation, the subconscious mind has devised various methods to spend that excess energy. It has us foot waving, pencil chewing, finger tapping, nail biting, twitching, blinking excessively, head jerking, and more. All of this is done in an effort to reduce the excessive energy levels of the body to normal or near-normal levels.

It is important to understand that if we have feelings of nervousness and apprehension and do not know why, it may not be psychological, but may be based on the simple fact that our chi levels are simply too high and many parts of us may simply be overactive as a result.

During acts of stroking, patting and petting, as well as through the natural open-gated subconscious mind psychic conduits existing between our pets and ourselves, our pet is drawing chi and simultaneously helping to reduce the excessive chi [when it exists], in our body to tolerable levels. This will not only help us on a daily basis but may actually extend our life spans.

DEFENSE AGAINS ANIMAL VAMPIRES

Generally, there is no need to defend ourselves against animal energetic vampirism since an animal's energetic needs, such as those of our pets, though constant, are small and normally harmless. However, if we ever find ourselves needing to defend against a professionally altered energy draining animal, we can do the following:

[1] The very first course of action for us to take is to physically separate ourselves from the animal.

[2] The second is to close our end of any subconscious mind psychic conduits that may be established between the animal and us.

Note: *A simple way to close the gate at our end of such a psychic conduit is to create and maintain in ourselves feelings of revulsion for the animal, pointing out in our mind anything about the animal that we find personally distasteful.*

[3] Then, of course, we could, as a last resort, kill the animal. However, this is a drastic step and we must be certain that the animal is, indeed, what we believe it to be.

Caution: *We must not allow our imaginations to run away with us by coloring and labeling an animal something that it isn't. That is, we must never allow a fanciful imagination to create in us a paranoia that may lead to the death of an innocent animal.*

PLANT VAMPIRES

Plants, even seemingly complex plants, require a great deal less energy than animals do in order to survive and flourish. And even though they too are constantly seeking chi, because their requirements are so minimal, their danger to us is generally minimal also. However, just as animals and inanimate objects can be used as chi-draining instruments that can be very dangerous or even fatal to us, plants can be used in the same way.

127

Fortunately, the use of plants in this manner lies well beyond the ability of the average occultist or psychic. Why? The reason is that plants are much too sensitive to any form of negativity, especially anything that they sense might harm them in any way. This means that they are quick to close their psychic gates at the very first sign of danger, which makes them, at best, rather difficult to work with as agents of foul play.

Even for many mystics, especially uninitiated mystics, the process would simply be much too time consuming and would require the sort of finesse lying parsecs beyond their present abilities. Any awkward attempt to use a plant in this manner, for example, would immediately send the plant into shock, which often results in the death of the plant. A dead plant does not, in the final analysis, make a viable intermediate and cannot help the psychic assailant in any way to achieve their end.

Because the energetic requirements of plants are so nominal and their use as cursed objects is difficult to achieve, we should not be concerned about having to defend ourselves from any member of the plant kingdom. Even so, if we suspect that we are the victims of a plant that seems to draw too much chi from us, we have two options: either to destroy the plant or to get professional help from a mystic qualified to deal with the specifics of the problem.

TELEPATHIC ATTACKS

What is a telepathic attack?

Simply, a telepathic attack consists of thoughts that are introduced into our mind by someone else.

Although, unquestionably, energetic vampiric attacks are the most prevalent assaults we face daily, telepathic attacks, being much more common than many of us think, run a close second. And just like energetic vampire attacks, they are taking place all around us every day in one form or another.

Most of them are relatively benign, innocuous, unintentional events that, in the scheme of things, have very little, if any real impact on our lives. Even so, in rare cases, there is the potential for harm. Others, however, are perpetrated by individuals who may target us intentionally and can, both in content and purpose, be quite sinister in nature. The latter can range from a brief, temporary, minor negative influence lasting only seconds, to something more extensive, lasting, perhaps, as long as the rest of our lives.

Minor attacks can result in nightmares, changes in attitudes, quirky behavior, unexplainable nervousness, unwarranted fears, and more. Some attacks, generated intentionally by those who have a command over the process, can be severe enough to cause a rapid decline in health, insanity, or even death.

What makes telepathic attacks so insidious in nature and often hard to detect is that whatever images or thoughts arise in the victim's conscious mind are generally accepted to be their own. That is, unless the victim has a great deal experience in this area, they would normally have no idea that the thought was established in their mind by another person. Clearly, this makes a telepathic attack, whether harmful or not, an egregious and unwanted invasion of privacy.

Even thoughts transferred during a minor telepathic attack can be quite disconcerting, especially if those thoughts are completely alien to our nature. The attack can, for example, consist of thoughts that involve injuring someone else, perhaps someone we love, or there may be thoughts of inflicting harm on ourselves, such as vagrant suicidal thoughts.

Even if those thoughts are not acted upon, they can certainly cause the victim great concern. In more severe cases, a telepathic attack can be, for all intents and purposes, tantamount to a subconscious mind psychic siege, where the victim is inundated with so many negative images over a protracted period of time that they begin to doubt their own sanity.

Although telepathic attacks can come at any time, there are times when we are most vulnerable, such as when we are either sleeping or just falling asleep. The reason for this is that during these periods, except while dreaming, the conscious mind is normally very quiet, virtually dormant, and so whatever telepathic images are sent through subconscious mind psychic conduits necessarily encounter little or no conscious mind resistance.

One of the telltale signs of a telepathic siege is the recurrence of the same nightmare. It does not necessarily have to take place on consecutive nights. In fact, it could be somewhat infrequent. The most likely reason for this repetition is that the psychic attacker probably lacks the skill necessary to vary the nature of the attack, and so there is a tendency to repeat the identical elements over and over again, and to inadvertently produce the same nightmare.

Even so, a nightmare is not necessarily the product of a telepathic attack. Many nightmares are nothing more than the result of some inner turmoil or stress, and are self-generated. Still, if we ever find ourselves subjected to the same nightmare on more than one occasion, even if there are minor variations in content or endurance, we may not necessarily be wrong in suspecting outside influences, and some sort of telepathic deviltry, may, in fact, be at work in our life.

Although subconscious mind psychic attacks are generally telepathic in nature, on rare occasions a subconscious mind psychic attack can be created clairvoyantly. This form of attack is much less frequent because it requires greater skill on the part of the attacker. Here, the psychic attacker clairvoyantly propels the victim headlong into another reality.

It could, for example, be the reality of someone in great physical distress, someone undergoing a tortuous disease, or even someone suffering insanity. An attacker adept at the process may even thrust their victim into the reality of something that is not human at all, perhaps that of an animal, such as a snake, mole, worm, hog, or even an insect. An insect? Yes. It does not take very much effort to imagine how nightmarishly distressing that could be - to be suddenly tossed into a world of such blind and utter savageness as that of the insect.

Fortunately, there are very few people that have that level of training, or the ability to bring this about, and so the odds of becoming the victim of such a dark and nefarious mystic are remote. But, then again not so remote that it could not happen.

Chapter 10: Some Closing Thoughts

Keep in mind that this course was designed as an advanced technical reference manual for those who have already studied our Chi Power Plus course and have built up a fair amount of energy. However, this program will work without the knowledge from Chi Power Plus, the difference is with the added benefit of understanding Chi Power Plus and our Advanced Chi DVD methods. When you combine the energy producing techiques contained in our Advanced Chi DVD and apply them to the techniques and concepts in this manual, you get a highly increased effectiveness of the techniques.

Respectfully,

A.Thomas Perhacs, Publisher

www.mindforcesecrets.com

www.advancedmindpower.com

www.chipower.com

My Other Products

Manipulation

Mind Force Hypnosis

Chi Power Plus

Mind Portal

Magneto

Power of the Mind

Closed Door Hypnosis Files

Advanced Chi DVD

Dim Mak Striking

The Goal Setting Formula

Chi Power Inner Circle Membership

Aknowledgements:

I think it goes without saying that when you put together a work as all encompassing as this one, there are a lot of people to thank. There is no way I can take credit for much of the information contained in this resource manual.

I've spent many years training with the very best and have put in the time to become privy to many of the closely guarded techniques in this book and know that I would be foolish to mention some of those who have taught me.

My wife Mary Jane puts up with my strange lifestyle of meditation and Chi Power Training, so I have to give her credit for allowing me the time to get my work done, even when I am still working deep into the early morning. I love her very much and appreciate all she does for me and my four children.

I would like to mention my four kids because over the years they have eached helped me in various ares of my business from writing up orders, burning cds and DVDs to making sure our customers were taking care of. Alex, Tommy, Samantha, and Camille, I love you all and appreciate all your help.

I would also like to aknowledge my business partner and friend Robin Jones, as he has taught me so many of the techniques contained in this guide. He and I have been through some things over the years, as it is inevitable when you commit to training the mind and body in ways that most people would never believe. I look forward to divulging more secrets (maybe) at a later date and time, so that others can get this esoteric information to work for them.

I would also like to thank all of the authors, writers and teachers that I have used as a basis for some of the concepts in this manuscript. They are too many to mention, but maybe some day I will take the time to catelog them all....

Enjoy this information and take it to heart. It works!

- Al Perhacs

CPSIA information can be obtained at www.ICGtesting.com
Printed in the USA
BVOW05s2041111113

336032BV00006B/80/P